Sex Roles and Aging:
Theory and Research from a Systems Perspective

Contributions to Human Development

Vol. 15

Series Editor
John A. Meacham, Buffalo, N.Y.

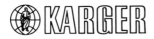

Basel · München · Paris · London · New York · New Delhi · Singapore · Tokyo · Sydney

Sex Roles and Aging: Theory and Research from a Systems Perspective

Jan D. Sinnott, Baltimore, Md., USA
With chapters by
Joan S. Rabin and *Michael T. Windle*

3 figures and 18 tables, 1986

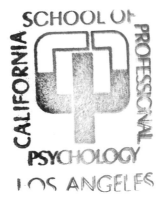

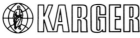

KARGER

Basel · München · Paris · London · New York · New Delhi · Singapore · Tokyo · Sydney

Contributions to Human Development

National Library of Medicine, Cataloging in Publication
    Sinnott, Jan D.
    Sex roles and aging: theory and research from a systems perspective/
    Jan D. Sinnott, with chapters by Joan S. Rabin and Michael T. Windle.
    – Basel; New York: Karger, 1986. –
    (Contributions to human development; vol. 15)
    Bibliography: p.
    Includes index.
    1. Aged – psychology 2. Identification (Psychology) – in old age I. Rabin, Joan S. II. Windle, Michael T.
    III. Title   IV. Series
    W1 CO778S v. 15 [HQ 1075 S617s]
    ISBN 3–8055–4207–0

©   Copyright 1986 by S. Karger AG, P.O. Box, CH-4009 Basel (Switzerland)
    Printed in Switzerland by Druckerei 'Der Bund', Berne (Switzerland)
    ISBN 3–8055–4207–0

Contents

Contents

Preface

In the brief time since the topics of sex roles and aging became important to psychologists, to researchers, and to the general public, considerable work on theory, measurement, and data collection has been completed. The purpose of this book is to consolidate this recent work on sex roles and aging, and to interpret what has been done. A further purpose is to suggest ways in which advances in other fields – fields as divergent as sociobiology, systems theory, cognitive psychology, and the so-called 'new' physics – can assist in the understanding of sex-role development in later life. This book, then, represents an attempt to bridge disciplines and areas within psychology and to suggest new directions in which we might proceed.

This book is written for students and teachers of human development, for researchers in development and aging, and for those who work with older adults and their families. The survey of recent work and the distillation of a set of 'ten commandments' for future research will be especially useful for the student or teacher who is attempting to become familiar with this knowledge area. Very little has been consolidated in this field, and sex-role development in adulthood is seldom discussed in general texts. The researcher (or potential researcher) can make use of the rich and varied theoretical perspectives described in the book and can be guided by those 'ten commandments'. He or she can also attend to the methodological issues raised in later chapters, a discussion which will help inform the interpretation made of sex-role development data.

Those who work with older adults and their families will be most interested in the several perspectives on the measuring of roles in later life. The possibility that roles are also manifestations of cognitive ability (as one theory would suggest) opens the possibility that role-related behavior could be developed into an assessment device for cognitive processes. The diverse views discussed also offer a rich source of ideas on roles for the general reader who will see support, in many places, for the social activist's stance that both types of sex-role behaviors should be valued and used by both sexes.

This book is unusual in providing a consolidation of recent work in mature adult sex-role development. It also reports details of a major study of sex-role development in older adults aged 60 and over. This book represents a first attempt to apply some new and complex models of life-span change over time to one area of development, sex-role development. Such new models include dialectics, 'new' physics paradigms, general systems theory paradigms, and ideas of biological adaptation. This book addresses the following topics: adaptation, adult development, aging, adrogyny, cognitive development, health, life experiences, mental health, methodology, problem solving, role conflict, sex roles, sociobiology, and systems theory.

One of the disappointments encountered by the author while preparing this work was the dearth of information on certain questions central to any understanding of sex-role development in late years. One of these questions, for example, concerned behavioral validation of reported roles. Longitudinal data were also lacking, but are essential to any understanding of behavioral *development,* i.e. behavioral change over time. Many other examples of gaps in knowledge can be found. Clearly any survey is limited by what other investigators have been able to do, but also must go beyond the information in hand to draw some conclusions and point the way toward future efforts. In this book there is an attempt – the reader is warned when this occurs – to stretch beyond references in hand and over gaps in information for the purpose of deriving larger concepts and theoretical points of departure.

The following is a brief outline of what is discussed in this book. The first focus of attention (chapter 1) is the historical background of studies in sex-role development in later adulthood and aging. The field appears to have been created as a result of interest in role development in general, interest in aging, focus on social change related to sex roles, creation of instruments to measure attitudes, and awareness of the dialectical interplay of social, biological, psychological, and behavioral forces in any single life story. These all played a part in the genesis of the field of life-span sex roles. Social-learning theory and cognitive-development theory are explored, along with biologically based approaches and anthropological information. The main ideas of the emerging life-span models are described; these include work by *Gutmann, Loevinger, Hefner, Garnets* and *Pleck.* The measurement of sex roles has gone from bipolar to bidimensional, with impact on theory. *Bem* has made important contributions here.

This brings us to the second section (chapter 2), which is focused on theories of sex-role development in later life. In it the most common approaches, mentioned above, are outlined and extended to late-life development. New approaches pertinent to late-life development are also described. These include: postformal, adult cognitive abilities which could underlie complex roles; general systems theory, which views roles as a process of handling information and energy within and between living systems which change over time; and dialectics, which treats roles as means of synthesizing various developmental dimensions.

Chapter 3 is focused on conceptualization of late-life sex-role development as an adaptation over time. This chapter was prepared by *Joan Rabin* of Towson State University, Maryland, who is responsible for much innovative thinking in this area. Adaptation and dependency are discussed, as are the value for survival of agency (stereotypical masculinity) and communion (stereotypical femininity).

Potential theoretical underpinnings are drawn from cognitive psychology, models of dynamic change, systems theory, general models of aging, sociobiology, physics, clinical psychology, humanistic personality theory, and theories of sex differences in chapter 4. That chapter, however, is entitled 'What Little We've Learned so Far' because, compared with what's needed, so little understanding has been developed. Studies discussed in this chapter address sex roles and the nature of masculinity and femininity, the influence of situational factors, well-being, self-concept, and models of change over time.

In chapter 5 data from several important studies of roles and aging of the last 5 years are presented. Some are published; others represent work underway. These studies focus on androgyny, its prevalence and correlates; sex-role learning and life events; well-being in old age; and age differences or age changes. The studies sometimes have conflicting results but overall suggest that developmental role changes might be occurring and that the context of roles and role responses matters. This chapter ends with ten important conclusions for sex-role research:

We must not jump to conclusions that responses on a scale will be predictive of behavior.

Responses to sex-role instruments do mean something.

Masculinity, femininity, and androgyny have been shown to be adaptive.

Sex roles are meaningful in terms of social expectations.

Sex roles are meaningful ways to organize one's sense of self as socially efficacious, to create a sense of personal conformity, and to organize self-concept.

The meaning of sex roles depends on age and developmental stage.

Models of sex-role changes over time can be of many types.

Sex-role complexity and later-life sex-role development may be linked to cognitive abilities such as postformal thought and problem-solving skills.

Sex-role developmental theory suggests 'new' physics concepts and might make use of them.

Sex-role development theory can make use of ideas in systems theory.

Chapters 6 through 8 include a report on a major study of sex roles in old age conducted by the author and funded by the National Institute on Aging, and incorporating some of the new thinking on roles described earlier in the book. We conducted a study of 364 community-dwelling mature adults, aged 60 and over, to determine: (1) whether they generally describe themselves in androgynous sex-role terms or in nonandrogynous terms; (2) whether current life-experiences, past milestone events, or perceived social expectations about roles might be related to described sex role, and (3) whether sex-role complexity is associated with successful aging. These research questions were embedded in a theoretical view of sex-role development in which the sex role adopted is adapted to the biological, psychological, social, and environmental contingencies experienced by the individual at a given life stage. Measures included the Bem Sex Role Inventory; standard assessments of verbal intelligence and mental health; measures of physical health, morale, and life-event stress; questions on milestone events, decision-making, and demographic data.

We determined that this cohort of older respondents was predominantly androgynous. The androgynous members experienced several recent life circumstances which differed from those of the masculine and feminine groups; some milestone events also seemed specific for the masculine versus feminine groups. Elders most often professed the sex role they believed society expected of them; those who professed a role different from social expectation usually had appropriately sex-typed expectations. On most measures the androgynous respondents aged most 'successfully', although not all the comparisons were significant.

Interpretation of these factors is carried out in chapter 9. Adults and society seem to adapt to each other's multidimensional systems over time. Five patterns of sex roles are important to consider:

(1) Androgynous, unconflicted. These women and men, scored androgynous, perceived that society expected them to be androgynous, and generally were not socialized to be stereotyped feminine or stereotyped masculine. Besides enjoying the generally positive aging of the androgynous group, they as a group would not be expected to suffer from conflict about their roles.

(2) Androgynous, conflicted. This group generally saw themselves as possessing a complex role, but experienced conflict about that role due to past milestone events, current life-situations, or perceived social expectations which seemed to reinforce them for displaying only one aspect of their complex role. This group would enjoy the advantages of androgyny (if their behavior matched that role) while possibly suffering from the effects of conflict.

(3) Appropriate sex-type (men – masculine; women – feminine), no conflict. These individuals appear to be reinforced for a traditional sex role, perceived such a role to be appropriate for them, and identified with that role. While the experience of aging appeared less positive overall for these persons, they did not suffer from conflict.

(4) Masculine/feminine; sex-type inappropriate, conflicted. These individuals described themselves in traditional role terms, but terms that did not match their biological sex. Those experiencing conflict between expectations, reinforcements, and identity would be expected to show the greatest strain, although persons with an inappropriate sex type are at risk of conflict under any circumstances.

(5) Undifferentiated. Apparently this was a group of complex individuals who may be beyond the androgynous stage (at some point of sex-role transcendence) or may never have identified with any sex role. Some appeared to suffer conflict. More work needs to be done to separate the adaptive and maladaptive subgroups here.

Methodological and statistical considerations are discussed in chapter 10 by *Michael Windle,* who is expert in developmental measurement issues and associated with the Johnson O'Connor Research Foundation in Chicago, Illinois. Questions have been raised as to the appropriateness of the Bem Sex-Role Inventory for older adults. Are the scores of older adults equivalent to those for younger ones? New confirmatory and exploratory factor-analytic techniques are used along with older factor-analytic strategies to obtain several answers to this question. The discussion that follows points out the limits of knowledge prior to the conduct of longitudinal studies. Chapter 11 contains suggestions as to the next steps we need to take to study sex roles adequately, including: a focus on context; behavior, in addition to reported attitudes; the impact of life events and transitions; gender-linked perceived expectations; role salience; awareness that all roles are implicitly related to some standard; belief systems; models employed; impact of roles on society; adaptivity; reporting style; methodology; and longitudinal research. 14 explicit suggestions are made.

The author acknowledges the crucial support received from the National Institute on Aging in the three forms of a Research Grant No. 2107 (which funded the study reported here), a Postdoctoral Fellowship, and (currently) acceptance as a Guest Scientist at the Gerontology Research Center (National Institute on Aging, National Institutes of Health), Learning and Problem Solving Section, Laboratory of Behavioral Sciences (Baltimore, Maryland). The support and ideas of *David Arenberg,* LPS Section Chief, immensely enriched this book. The creativity and analytical skills of *Leonard Giambra* (GRC, NIA) were an important stimulus to improvement during the author's preparation of this book.

The support staff at the Gerontology Research Center were very helpful, with special thanks to *Susan Robinson,* who analyzed data, *Judy L. Friz* and *Barbara S. Hiscock* who proofed, and *Ann Brown, Rita Wolferman,* and *Robin Armstrong* who typed the manuscript. Thanks are due to Towson State University, Maryland, for its support of the project, especially to the secretarial staff of the Psychology Department, and to *Sandra Kafka* who assisted in the survey of literature. The University of Maryland, especially the Center on Aging, deserves gratitude for supporting the proposal for the study in chapters 6 through 9, and for administrative support during the term of the project.

Special thanks are due to *Jody Olsen, Jean Grambs, Marilyn Block, Jan Davidson, Cathy Gaddy, Suzanne Sedge, Colleen Royce,* and the team of interviewers, all of whom played crucial roles in the project. A thousand thanks to the Baltimore County Department on Aging and to the directors and staff of their senior centers who put us in touch with so many interesting respondents. A 'thank you' also to those respondents themselves. The many, many reviewers and colleagues who commented on parts or all of this work deserve thanks for their help in sharpening ideas and extending dialogue. I am grateful to my many colleagues in physics, clinical practice, biology, brain research, systems theory, and humanist psychology who challenged my original ideas sufficiently to allow me to become aware of the general patterns underlying all these fields. Colleagues associated with the Institutes run by *Jean Houston* have been especially helpful in my reaching a new level of awareness about these developmental patterns common to many domains. Gratitude is due to The Gerontological Society of America, publisher of *The Gerontologist* and the *Journal of Gerontology,* for their permission to reprint portions of my articles [*Sinnott, 1977, 1982; Windle and Sinnott, 1985*].

Finally, many thanks to my friends and to my family, all of whom supported me through this portion of the path of my development. One of my goals in offering this book is to give them, and my larger human family, a greater chance to know – and live – a richer 'self'. This self may have many more possibilities and a lifetime with potential far more interesting than our current dreams would even suggest. This potential can come to life through greater awareness of how we behave, why we behave, how we change, and how our local behavior might interact with the larger events of which we are a creative part.

1. The Evolution of Sex-Role Theory: Life-Span Development

Conceptualizations of sex roles have been a function of philosophy, history, economics, and politics. Awareness that sex roles exist, and are influential, and that this occurs at all times in life, has also been a function of those four forces. These influences quietly shape the choice of problems to investigate and research projects to pursue. Between paradigm shifts, such as those discussed by *Kuhn* [1962], most scientists in a given field accept some view of the world that dominates their field and choose problems accordingly [*Bachrach*, 1982]. This world view is driven by the needs of the times, be they ideational, economic, population, or political needs [*Guttentag and Secord*, 1983; *Riegel*, 1973]. Driven by a need for cognitive consistency, individuals adopt the new view as 'natural'. In a world at war, for example, the role of a man is seen as that of a warrior and the role of a woman becomes that of a worker/mother; after a return to peace, the woman may be constrained within the role of mother while the now suddenly 'nonwarlike' male is redefined as worker. Theories of adjustment, development, and mental health are quick to conform to the demands of the belief system and the historical situation. What is healthy, natural role behavior one day is maladaptive and unnatural the next. Social psychology has made it clear that even radical shifts in ideas and behavior are accepted to maintain consistency in a system, provided motivation is high enough. Researchers in human development are not immune to these general laws. We study what seems important at the time.

These processes have been active in forming research on sex-role development, and in directing our attention now to sex-role development in old age. The main philosophical/practical changes which brought about and influenced the study of sex-role development in maturity included greater longevity, awareness of dialectical, systems theory and relativistic ways of viewing reality, population increases, movements for social change, and social equity, changing demands of childbearing and work roles in Western culture, sophistication in awareness of biological and psychological processes, and rapid change in role demands coupled with a breakdown in the usefulness of traditional behavior. Greater longevity ensured that there were enough older persons around to be observed. It also guaranteed that a larger proportion of the population would be beyond childbearing age, beyond the traditional demands of the parental imperative [Gutmann, 1975, 1985]. These persons would be exploring nontraditional ways of adopting roles in society because they would of necessity have few models to follow.

Population increases freed both women and men from the need to concentrate their attention on childbearing and childrearing, and gave both sexes the chance to consider the other activities that might fill their time. Movements for social change and social equity, resulting from political and economic changes in Western societies, pointedly brought home the fact that everyday situations could be different. Role-related designations were seen to be value-laden, political, and somewhat arbitrary. If one or the other of these role distinctions and behaviors could be changed, perhaps many of them could. A search began to find intrinsic meaning and utility for roles or to discard useless roles. That search eventually focused on both early and later life.

The awareness of dialectics, relativity, systems theory, and the world view of the so-called 'new' physics, all rising in prominence in the 20th century [see Wolf, 1981, for an overview], also had an impact on views of later life sex-role development. A dialectical viewpoint [Riegel, 1973] suggested that the polarity of divergent masculine and feminine roles could be expected to be resolved in a synthesis of some sort, a combined role. A relativistic world-view suggested that one was not concretely and forever the owner of certain concrete attributes but, rather, that one was only more or less something in relation to another. In the new physics, standards were not absolute and the nature of a system was found to depend upon the point of view of the observer. Systems theory [von Bertalanfy, 1968; Miller, 1978] suggests that social systems tend to perpetuate themselves for the sake of continuity and that some given set of social roles may not be the best way to structure power in a changing society. New demands call for new forms to serve old needs.

Meanwhile, the nature of work in Western societies was changing. Differences in musculature between women and men and changes in childbearing capabilities were no longer issues in assigning work roles or, therefore, sex roles. These rapid changes necessitated new everyday survival skills, which meant that traditions regarding roles were less valued as time went on, perhaps because they were less useful. Changes in the nature of work were linked with the growth of knowledge and technology. As sophistication in awareness of physical and mental processes occurred it became difficult to argue that roles were based on immutable biological differences. The result of all these changes and processes was a philosophical shift in regard to role concepts and concepts about the nature of the person. The result for research was a focus on role changes over time, where such a focus had never been considered before.

Sex-Role Concepts: Developmental Theory

Looking more closely at specific sex-role theories, we see how these have evolved. Early views of sex-role development focused upon masculine and feminine roles as biologically based and, once established in childhood, consistent throughout the life span [*Shields,* 1975; *Tavris and Offir,* 1977]. The testing movement provided the impetus to quantify and validate such views. Masculinity and femininity were conceptualized as marking the two extreme endpoints of a continuum (fig. 1). Individuals were assumed to be optimally well-adjusted if their biological sex and their sex-role identity were the same. An individual who deviated from a prescribed sex role was seen as one whose psychosexual development was inadequate, rather than as a person who was flexible in meeting changing environmental demands. This view reflected the Freudian [*Freud,* 1905, 1925] approach which depicted sex-role identification in terms of resolution of the Oedipal conflict. Such a resolution involved the identification of a boy with his father and the girl, in a somewhat more circuitous way, with her mother. The possible learned nature of sex roles came to the forefront with the advent of social-learning theory, cognitive-developmental theory, biologically oriented inquiries, anthropological investigation, and the life-span approach.

Social Learning Theory. Whereas *Freud* and other functionalists implied that sex roles merely unfold out of an innate potential, the social-learning theorists [*Bandura and Walters,* 1963; *Mischel,* 1970] posited that such roles were learned via imitation and observation of parents and other adult models. Reinforcement then led to the establishment of behavioral patterns. Although changes in reinforcement contingencies

Traditional-polarized roles
in differentiated persons,
may be a 'given' in nature, or
may be learned

Bem – role continuum in
differentiated persons

Bem (revised) –
differentiated versus
undifferentiated persons

Hefner et al. –
developmental progression,
'beyond' sex roles;
incorporates cognitive
elements

Garnets and Pleck –
norms versus perceived roles
and role salience;
incorporates evaluative
self-concept

Riegel – role behavior is a
result of synthesis of both
individual multidimensional
development and situational
demands

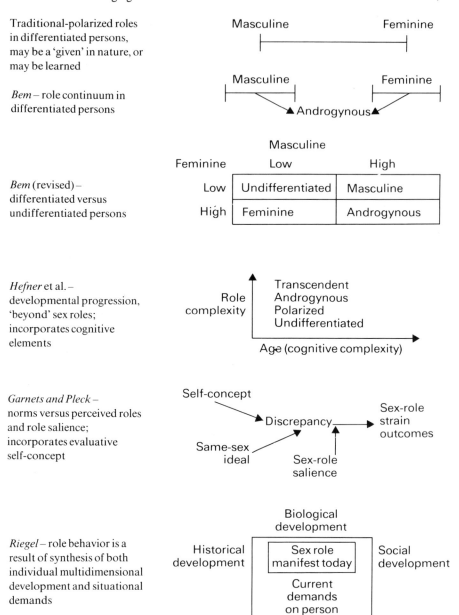

Fig. 1. Evolution of concepts of the development of sex-role identity.

allowed the possibility for sex-role change, it was assumed that the sex-typed roles which were reinforced did not change significantly during one's life span. Modeling the behaviors of the same sex was thought to begin at a very early age and to be reinforced into adulthood. *Mischel* [1970], for example, stated that 'boys do not learn baseball by watching girls and girls do not learn about fashions from observing boys'. However, research that has focused on modeling of adult behavior or global personality traits shared by parent and child has *not* found that children closely follow the behavior or personality of the same-sex adult [*Maccoby and Jacklin,* 1974].

Cognitive-Developmental Theory. The cognitive-developmental approach [*Kohlberg,* 1966; *Piaget,* 1948] impacted further on the learned nature of sex roles. The child's perception of sex-role identification was thought to precede sex-appropriate behavior; i.e. the child discovered that two sexes existed, thought about himself or herself as being a boy or a girl, considered differences between the sexes, and came to some fairly stable notions as to what 'boy-man' versus 'girl-woman' connoted. Some of the same behavioral factors that the social-learning theorists proposed were also expected, except that cognitive identification with a same-sex parent preceded the modeling of behaviors in terms of observation and imitation. This approach increased awareness of the child's cognitive development and its impact upon sex-role identity. The cognitive-developmentalists also assumed that both children and adults maintained a relatively consistent concept of themselves as male or female, and that the search for congruence between beliefs and behavior led to the maintenance of appropriate roles. This view may be contrasted with the social-learning view in which reward is the key to the persistence of sex-appropriate behavior. Both theoretical viewpoints, however, emphasize the establishment of such an identity early in life with consistency assumed in adulthood as well.

Biologically Based Inquiries. The learning perspective on sex roles has also received a valuable contribution from the biological perspective of *Money and Ehrhardt* [1972]. These researchers have studied children who genetically, and on the basis of prenatal hormones, would have been expected to develop the gender identity of one sex but because of mishap (for example, structural damage or deformity of the genitals) were assigned to the opposite sex. Interview data collected from the families of such children indicated that seeming acceptance of the assigned sex- and gender-role identity development proceeded commensurate with the child's acceptance of assigned gender identity. While these studies are by no means conclusive, they do point out the overwhelming impact of socialization.

Anthropological Investigation. Anthropological study has yielded additional interesting support for the learned nature of sex roles and has led to questioning the implicit notion of consistent, appropriate behaviors for each gender. The large impact of culture on any given society's notion of what is appropriate male and female behavior has been exemplified by *Mead's* [1935] comparison of three primitive societies. Both the men and women of the Arapesh tribe were described as being passive, nurturant, cooperative, and sensitive, traits perceived as feminine in American culture. The Mundugamore men and women were characterized as aggressive, suspicious, and uncaring, traits perceived as masculine in American culture. The Tchambuli men behaved in ways our society typically defines as feminine while the women exhibited what we might define as stereotypically masculine traits. The importance of culture-specific specialization has been expounded in numerous articles and books with respect to more modern societies as well [*Deaux,* 1976; *Frieze,* et al. 1978; *Tavris and Offir,* 1977].

The anthropological perspective has been used by researchers to explore the function of sex-roles in terms of survival of the species [*Gutmann,* 1975]. Cultural universals are presumed to reflect basic human propensities; their consistency is assumed to be of some importance in terms of survival. Proponents of the learning approach, which emphasizes socialization,view exceptions to cultural universals as evidence for the greater impact of environment on heredity. Opponents point out that a few exceptions do not make a case against biological mechanisms but rather show evolutionary change based upon some special environmental conditions.

One such cultural universal is division of labor. *Gutmann* [1975, 1985] suggested divisions of labor based on the parental imperative, i.e. the demands of childrearing. *Frieze* et al. [1978] have presented an interesting account of relevant anthropological research from this perspective. They point out that sex is employed in almost all cultures as one criterion for dividing family responsibilities. Cross-culturally, large, extended family structures show more sex-role differentiation than small, nuclear, mobile family units such as those that predominate in the USA today [*Barry* et al., 1957]. In primitive, less complex cultures than ours, women perform childbearing and support functions, while the typically larger and more muscular men, who are never at a physical disadvantage due to pregnancy and are not needed for nursing, leave the home to wage battle and retrieve food.

Role differentiation in the past seemed to serve the practical purposes of contributing to the continued survival of the group and coping with particular environmental demands. Our societal needs do not now include constant childbearing because overpopulation is our current problem. Today, almost every role requirement previously filled by one sex to the exclusion of the other can now be shared by either sex. With very obvious exceptions such as bearing a child and nursing it if desired, men and women can share in all aspects of work and of childrearing and socialization and have begun to do so increasingly [*Albrecht* et al., 1979; *Araji*, 1977]. Women have increasingly moved into the work force and are sharing the historically male-dominated provider role. Thus, both sexes have greater flexibility to pursue a wider range of experiences.

Life-Span Approach

The life-span approach to sex-role development has been a relatively recent phenomenon. *Neugarten* [1964], *Gutmann* [1975], and *Block* [1973] explored changes in male and female role expectations during adulthood that were based upon social expectation and major developmental tasks. These studies will be discussed in more detail in a later section. *Block* [1973] and *Riegel* [1973] viewed the manifestation of cultural sex roles as a function not only of biological demands and past learning experiences, but of the nature of economic systems, the historical moment, and the philosophical system within which they are defined (fig. 1). Thus, sex roles in this perspective imply dynamic change based upon the individual and the social and cultural climate.

Loevinger's [1977] milestones of ego development and their extrapolations to sex-role development form the basis of *Block's* [1973] approach. In the earliest period, the main developmental concerns of the child are genderless, and identity constitutes a mere naming of gender: 'I am a boy/girl.' Later, conformity to learned patterns becomes the main task; this is reflected in the development of sex-role stereotypes and sex-role bifurcation. The conformist stage is followed by one of self-criticism based on comparison with an abstract ideal, thereby moderating the stereotypical role. With the advent of autonomy, individualization results as conflicts, aroused during the conformity and conscientious stages, are resolved. At this point, differentiation of sex role is said to occur. The highest, most integrated level of functioning finds the individual evolving a complex identity which combines aspiration, experience, and previously polarized traits. In sex-role terms, this period is one of androgyny.

Hefner et al. [1975] have proposed a life-span approach to the development of sex-role identity. Their hierarchical stages include: (1) global, undifferentiated sex roles; (2) polarized, or traditional masculine/feminine roles, and (3) transcendent roles which combine both masculinity and femininity. While the young child most likely has not defined a sex role, and the adolescent most likely has overdefined it, the adult synthesizes roles into more complex wholes (fig. 1). For individuals who have 'transcended' masculinity and femininity, psychological adjustment is no longer tied to these dichotomous sets of traits, even as in the blend of androgyny. Unfortunately, the measurement of 'transcendence' as distinct from androgyny has not yet been fully operationalized. *Garnets and Pleck* [1979] have begun this task with their concept of sex-role salience that is currently under empirical scrutiny.

Garnets and Pleck [1979] have presented the most recent conceptual analysis on the basis of sex-role strain analysis. Their viewpoint combines social-learning and life-span development. They feel that the ultimate harm of traditional sex roles is the devaluation an individual may experience if he or she does not conform to traditional standards set by sex-role norms. Thus, strain results from discrepancy between the individual's self-perception and his or her perceptions of social expectations. *Garnets and Pleck* also measure the degree of salience of sex-role characteristics for the individual. The dichotomy of 'masculine' versus 'feminine' may not be an equally important distinction to everyone. Thus, the salience or importance of sex-role characteristics as a filter through which the individual views his or her behavior is measured. By combining measures of the individual's 'real' self-concept, same-sex 'ideal', and degree of sex-role salience, *Garnets and Pleck* propose two derived variables of real versus ideal discrepancy and sex-role strain outcome (fig. 1). As in *Bem's* [1979] conception, the long-run developmental trend is toward reduced sex-role salience.

Measurement of Sex Roles

Important methodological changes have occurred in conceptualizations of the measurement of sex roles. Whereas sex roles were traditionally defined in a bipolar sense, recent models of sex-role development view sex roles as bidimensional (fig. 1). *Bem* [1974] proposed that measurement be undertaken of 'androgyny'. Androgyny epitomizes the combination of both positive masculine and positive feminine traits in a single individual. Contrary to the traditional view that cross-typed behavior is aberrant, the current perception is that an increased behavioral repertoire including both traditionally masculine and feminine traits allows for greater situational flexibility and shows better adaptation. Under particular circumstances, 'feminine' behaviors might offer the best response to a situation, while under other circumstances, the most adaptive response for the same individual might involve 'masculine' behaviors. In combination with the complementary life-span approach, the optimally functioning individual would possess a wider array of behaviors to employ in adapting to different environmental and age demands. A large body of research has accumulated in support of more flexible and adaptive functioning by androgynous individuals [*Bem,* 1975; *Bem and Lenney,* 1976; *Bem* et al., 1976; *La France and Carmen,* 1980; *Sinnott,* 1977; *Spence* et al., 1975].

Bem [1974] was not the first to suggest the importance of integrating masculine and feminine behaviors. *Bakan* [1966] described two analagous role modalities – agency and communion – and their eventual integration. Agency is defined as self-assertion and self-expression, while communion involves a sense of oneness with a larger whole or others. Integration of these two disparate roles is the mature individual's fundamental task. *Jung* [1933], too, included the archetypes of animus (male) and anima (female) as important constructs held by each individual. Ignorance of one or the other was felt by *Jung* to be detrimental to the individual's full realization of self. He suggested that aging men could discover and acknowledge their tenderness and that aging women would become aware of and use their sharpness of mind. *Parson and Bales* [1955] found similar constructs in their dimensions of expressiveness and instrumentality. *Erikson* [1963] described inner and outer space orientations of females and males, respectively, with eventual synthesis in adulthood.

Bem [1974] was the first to introduce a single construct implying

positively valued 'masculine' and 'feminine' behaviors in an operationalized approach. *Constantinople* [1973] presented a critique of previous sex-role inventories, and *Bem* [1974] provided the beginning of a
fresh, new approach with her *Bem* Sex-Role Inventory (BSRI). (This is
discussed in more detail later in chapter 10.) Previous masculinity-femininity scales had treated the two as a single continuum, while *Bem*
provided for two orthogonal dimensions. Also, whereas femininity in the
past had been described as an absence of masculinity, *Bem* presented
both as separate compilations of positive characteristics.

In summary, conceptualizations of sex roles have been a function of
philosophy, history, economics, and politics. Researchers study what
seems important at the time. Roles have been conceptualized as
developing or unfolding, as learned via social encounters, or as enacted
after cognitive assimilation of a role concept in childhood. The relatively
recent life-span approach incorporates all of the above dimensions.
Measures of masculine and feminine roles have reflected the transition
from seeing roles as general concrete entities on a single continuum to
thinking of them as multicaused multifactor concepts of certain salience
at some life-span point.

2. Sex Roles in Context:
Cognitive, Dialectical, and Systems Views

Ideas about sex roles and sex-role development have been linked to ideas and advances in other aspects of science. In this chapter, three recent approaches to conceptualizing life-span sex-role development are presented. They all involve an examination of the *context* in which roles serve individuals, and an analysis of the ways in which the social system and the individual system interact to their mutual benefit. The first new approach is a consideration of how adult cognitive development (Piagetian formal and postformal operations, relativistic thought, awareness of necessary but subjective belief systems) might cause mature adults to know roles differently and therefore behave differently. The second new approach is an application of dialectical theory to suggest how roles might emerge and change over time as they reflect resolutions of developmental conflicts between biological, psychological, social, and historical dimensions of life. The third new approach is an application of systems theory to role development, considering roles as the intersections of two living systems, that of the organism and that of society. These three approaches are used (in chapters 5 and 11) to interpret what we know now about life-span sex-role development and to suggest future research directions (chapter 11).

Piagetian Formal and Postformal Thinking:
Adult Cognitive Development and Sex-Role Concepts

A number of investigators have recently addressed the topic of 'postformal' operations, i.e. those structures of thought which are a stage more complex in organization than *Piaget's* formal operations. Theories of postformal operations are presented in *Commons* et al. [1984], a book which compiles presentations from the First Harvard Symposium on Postformal Operations. A review by *Kramer* [1983] contains summaries and critiques of the various postformal positions and of the idea of post-formal operations. More work on postformal, mature adult thought is being done, possibly since the idea of cognitive development beyond adolescence is an appealing one. The question of interest here is: How might formal and postformal operations be related to a life-span model of sex-role development? To address this question it is necessary to examine some aspects of postformal operations and the argument itself more closely.

What kind of case is being made for a relation between cognitive development, especially formal and postformal operations, and sex roles? To oversimplify, it is the same type of case that *Kohlberg* [1966] makes about cognitive development and early sex-role development and about cognitive and moral development. Social relations, of which sex roles and moral development are examples, may be seen as based upon cognitive skills. As cognitive skills develop, the social relations can be understood and can become more complex, too. At those times, when the world can be known in a manner more complex than an abstract, formal one, roles also might be known in a way that is more complex. Having thought of the role in a complex way, one could then live it in a complex way.

How would roles be known in postformal terms? To answer this question, one must look at theories of postformal operations. According to *Kramer* [1983], authors of these theories all state that postformal thought is: (1) a distinct stage; (2) which subsumes formal operations, and (3) which incorporates a relativistic view of truth. Generally, then, a postformal cognitive stage could underlie a view of sex roles in which roles are not absolute but are created relative to the actor, i.e. with a subjective component. Some given formal structure of roles would be consciously chosen based on some belief system that is a subjective view of 'truth', from among a number of formal role structures. Further, what constitutes a given role, e.g. 'masculinity', would be known to be somewhat arbitrary and based partly on the perceiver's own experiences and resultant ideas of truth. Things are what they are only within a particular system [*von Bertalanffy,* 1968]. The postformal concept of sex roles, then, includes a necessary subjectivity. It operates by laws like those of the 'new' physics [*Sinnott,* 1981, 1983].

In a personal context, the role taken, or the role which one perceives that another takes, becomes what is agreed on by the persons in the interaction. The 'truth' of the role is therefore determined by a system of beliefs held by the persons in the interaction. Those persons in the interaction may even be aware that all roles are potentially available for them and that they are the ones to call the shots and decide what a given set of behaviors means in role terms. The individual is not in a roleless, undefined state, nor in possession of an absolute unchanging role, which is a permanent descriptor of one's identity, but rather is constantly, perhaps even consciously, creating a flexible role defined *in relation to* individuals and circumstances in one's context [*Sinnott,* 1978]. The last is a shared but also dually created perception of reality. In the framework of *Kelly's* [1955] theory of personality, persons are always moving to new 'places' where they must construct a new social meaning for the self in the context of evolving social structures within a given society's institutions. From the standpoint of sociobiological theory [*Lumsden and Wilson,* 1981], human social behaviors which have evolutionary use are possible because a cognitive filter permits them. Genes, in turn, control the type of cognitive filter which occurs. If potentially postformal cognitive filters are adaptive, then we would see more and more societies where adult sex roles are relativistic and flexible, which seems to be the case.

Role behaviors also may be seen as attempts to solve everyday life problems. Individuals learn to act in a way which helps them meet their goals. In the context of problem solving, postformal thought-based roles might permit greater creativity in using strategies to solve problems where the goal is unclear. Most everyday problems fall into that category [*Wood,* 1983]. The individual has the cognitive freedom to jump out of the system [*Hofstadter,* 1979] to some metalevel, make a decision about the rules of the game (i.e. which roles constitute his or her goals today and, therefore, which goals are appropriate), and jump back into the processing system to continue the work of solving the particular problem. For the postformal problem solver the solution to a problem may be in reaching a metagoal, namely the creation of a *process* which usually works in many systems in spite of widely varying sets of rules or belief systems. The adult postformal operational problem solver who is attempting to solve the problem of how to act in a sex-role-related situation in which the goal is unclear can: (1) jump out of the system to a higher level; (2) decide which belief/rule system (related to sex roles) to use; (3) jump back in and operate within that system of 'masculinity', 'femininity'; (4) test the results of that problem-solving attempt; (5) reinforce the use of the 'good process' (which is in step 2), and (6) continue living using this sort of metasolution for problems of this type.

These possibilities may be put into more concrete terms. Consider this scenario. A 40-year-old woman who lost her husband to cancer some months ago is noticing that her house needs an exterior paint job. She knows from her childhood training and her neighbors' behavior that it is not considered feminine to paint the house herself, although her gentle, feminine mother once did so for the sake of the family. She knows that the money for that job would be better spent for herself and the children's needs. She dislikes the immensity of the task, but she likes working outside with her hands for a change since her usual job requires only mental activity. If she does the paint job, will she be taking over her late husband's masculine role? Should she do the job?

Thinking about the scenario in a personal framework, we notice that the woman and her husband and the woman and her neighbors had apparently agreed together that painting the house was 'masculine', while she and her mother defined the same behavior as nurturing and 'feminine'. Thinking of her own needs and likes, and the needs of her children, she realized that it is not clear whether what she has thought about doing is more instrumental or more nurturant, more 'masculine' or more 'feminine'. It seems to be both. She decides that if she is ever to do anything she must step back from the situation (use postformal logical operations), choose a behavior based on a chosen belief system about truth (belief system = 'be pragmatic'), call it acceptably 'feminine' in terms of her own ('feminine') self-image, and act. She has faced the fact that this knowledge is partly subjective, has chosen to know in a certain way, and has let it influence her action.

Thinking about the scenario in problem-solving terms, the woman seems to have a clear subgoal – getting the house painted – but a fuzzy larger goal – keeping a coherent self-image. She therefore 'jumps out' of the system to a higher metalevel, and decides that the most important thing is to do *something*. That means dealing with the potential relativity of the self-image by making a decision as to what is 'feminine' for her, in relation to this situation and in view of her past history. The next step was to jump back into the problem-solving system, decide that she was still 'feminine' in this situation if she painted the house since it was also nurturant behavior and felt a little like a hobby. She tested the workability of this solution on several neighbors and one of her children, and they did not respond in a way that threatened her self-image. Pleased with the results, she filed the process away as a 'good process' to be used again later.

Thinking about the scenario in terms of the evolution of society, decisions such as that of this woman, multiplied over many individuals and occasions, could change the nature of concepts of 'femininity' and 'masculinity'. Simple awareness that sex roles are relative would also have that effect. The current phenomena we are witnessing as society considers questions of equity between the sexes attest to the fact that when individuals are aware that roles are not fixed by some natural law, individuals permit themselves role flexibility.

Systems Theory and Life-Span Roles

Systems theory is a theory of interacting processes and the way they influence each other over time to permit the continuity of some larger whole. Systems act so as to continue. Systems change because their own balances are not optimal or because they are influenced by other systems. Some authors who provide excellent descriptions of these general ideas are *von Bertalanffy* [1968], *Buckley* [1968], *Hofstadter* [1979], and *Miller* [1978]. *Miller's* discussion of living systems is especially useful to consider for a discussion of roles. Individuals, societies, and cells all appear to use similar processes to create boundaries, to take in stimulation, to process information, to act, and to change. For example, information is handled by cells, persons, and societies. For cells, information may be chemical and may be filtered by cell walls; for persons, information may be conceptual and may be filtered by perceptions; for societies information may be news and be filtered by censors. Cells, persons, and societies all exist in relation to each other. For example, a liver cell could not have formed into a liver cell without the feedback of the body, and a child who speaks English could not be that without the feedback of a culture. The liver cell exposed to carcinogens by the person system hosting it (and indirectly by the social system producing those substances) is influenced. The production of the carcinogen may keep the social living system healthy, but kill the cell system and the person system. Within systems theory, roles are structures of the social system which are equivalent to organs in the physical/person system; they are organized ways of ensuring that some vital function is performed.

As living systems – be they cell, person, or society – develop and age, they appear to proceed through a regular set of stages. They begin in disorder, that is, with a few parts concrete and defined. They become more orderly, defined, and bounded over time. They become overordered, overbounded, and mechanical or rigid before they disintegrate into disorder/new order. For example, early embryonic tissue is largely potential, able to be changed into a number of different cell/organ types. This flexibility without structure is gradually transformed into a state of some structure (e.g. organs) and some flexibility (e.g. ability to repair and regenerate tissue). Later in development some organs cannot regenerate any longer since tissues are too differentiated. In senescence all flexibility has been lost and any damage leads to deterioration and disintegration/death. When we move to the psychological realm we see series of these 'deaths' as persons pass from one state to another, suffering disorder in between, then reordering at a more complex level. Notice that the manner of change described here so briefly is similar in form to the ideas of *Prigogene* [1980] and the principles of entropy articulated in the so-called 'new' physics [*Prigogene and Stengers,* 1984].

Living systems which survive for any period of time contain many potential orders of complexity. The later orders are contained as 'seeds' in the earlier orders. An example is the more complex order of adolescence contained implicitly in the earlier forms of childhood. Systems which survive also contain a process by which the new can replace the old. Resistance to the emerging change means eventual massive harm – or death – to the system. Systems set up for change are said to be in a ready state, as opposed to the usual dynamic/steady state, or the terminal steady state. Systems that survive monitor their change processes to ensure continuity while change is permitted. They also are therefore flexible enough to adapt to many contexts. They can interface with many other systems without being engulfed or walling off valuable information from the other systems. The degree of order necessary to a system to keep it going is individual for the system.

How does this relate to sex-role development over the life span? Consider the person and society as living systems, each seeking continuity and meeting survival needs. These needs include control of information and energy flow. Sex roles are ways person and social systems can regulate the flow of information and energy (effort) between these while taking care of survival needs. The early stages of these systems are disordered in regard to roles, i.e. no roles are apparent. For example, the newborn is sex roleless, and a group of strangers is roleless. Later stages are associated with more concretized roles; in the person and in the group, masculinity and femininity may emerge. Final stages find the roles rigid and inflexible, so they would fail to respond to the pull of new needs. This failure of response leads to disorder and a search for new, more complex order. Systems theory suggests that this may be the transition we are seeing now in society and after the reproductive period and parental imperative [*Gutmann*, 1975] in each developing person. Rigid roles in the presence of new demands might lead to more complex integrations of role-related behaviors.

Systems theory leads to suggestions for the conceptualization of aging in general, and therefore for the understanding of sex-role development in older adults. The life course in systems terms might be thought of as three phases: youth involves personal expansion and definition; mature adulthood involves interactions with other systems while improving existing structure; and decline involves imposition of personal order irrespective of fit. In youth, data gathering is a major activity, cognition grows to the level of abstraction, energy is plentiful, breaking away and learning about the world are main developmental demands, and the system is driven less by preconception and more by events of the moment, which often include social learning. This would be a period of rigid roles. In maturity, energy and memory are less available and partly committed to already existing structures. Thought is practical and contextual as well as abstract and is determined by both past structures of thought and present incoming data. Demands are for interface with other systems, which increases differentiation. This would be an age for complex roles. In decline (not 'old age' but 'decline') energy is lacking and the easiest way to orient the system is 'top down', i.e. using the structures already available to make sense of everything, whether they fit or not. Roles at this point would be idiosyncratic representations of the last stage of role development of the organism before energy diminished so much that flexibility was lost. Interface with other systems would be avoided at this time and boundaries hardened defensively.

This general summary may give a flavor for the multifaceted causes, effects, and processes – all related to roles – stemming from the need for system continuity and intersystem interfaces. The reader is urged to look at the 'new' physics literature and systems literature mentioned earlier [e.g. *Wolf*, 1981] for more detailed and technical information.

A Dialectical Model[1]

Kline [1975], writing in *The Gerontologist,* made several well-docu-
mented points about the existence of role inconstancy during the life
span of women. She hypothesized that it may be this very inconstancy of
roles which accounts for women's relative resilience during the role
changes of old age. I would like to offer a reply to her article, not to challenge it, but to extend her hypothesis. *Kline* suggested that women are
subjected to repeated role discontinuities and learn to adjust to them,
thereby learning to adjust to the discontinuities of aging, too. I would
like to suggest, based on a review of the data of others, that a person's
ability to show *life-span variations in sex roles* is an indication of a general
flexibility which is associated in some way with more successful aging
and a longer life span.

There appear to be three possible explanations for this association.
First, general survival of the fittest may be the operant dynamic, and the
flexible person may also be one of the fittest. Second, it may be that the
generally creative and adaptive person survives, and that sex-role flexibility is but one form of that creativity. Finally, it is possible that the biological, psychological, and cultural tasks and expectations conflict for
the older adult; therefore, the older adult who is able to make a
behavioral synthesis, compromising among these factors, is more likely
to survive. I expect that the third explanation will prove to be the most
useful and that a thesis-antithesis-synthesis model [*Riegel,* 1976] holds
for the relationship between sex-role flexibility and successful aging. I
also believe, with *Bem* [1975], that the ability to synthesize disparate
roles, when the need arises, is an indicator of a general flexibility, adaptivity, or intelligent behavior, which in turn is related to successful aging.

Biological, Cultural, and Psychological Tasks of Older Adults
Today we are willing to ask a complex question: What is the function
of sex-role behaviors in the adaptation of the species, as well as in the
psychological functioning of the individual [*Block,* 1973; *Emmerich,*
1973]? From observation, experience, introspection, interviews, and
social indicators, it appears that the chief biological and psychological
tasks in old age are to maintain health, to continue to grow, and to
achieve integrity [*Erikson,* 1963]. From a cultural point of view, the old

---

[1] Reprinted from *Sinnott* [1977] by permission of *The Gerontologist.*

individual has a function larger than that of continuing and enhancing his or her own life, and that is to carry on the culture of the group [*de Beauvoir,* 1973].

This last task was a particularly important function when customs were transmitted orally, and social change was slow. When the older adult's wisdom was coupled with the power of seniority, it saved the individual from a loss of status with the decline of his or her physical abilities. It reduced the conflict between biological and social status. The role or tradition maintained might have little to do with the actual biological or psychological need of the old individual involved. It represented a past value investment, resulting from youthful choices which were once meaningful, and from a reduction of the conflict engendered when a physically less productive group member remains alive.

Sex roles seem to be a category of traditions maintained by the old individual in spite of their general lack of relevance. The elder might counsel young males to be aggressive and young females to be submissive because such counsel is consonant with the elder's previous behavior, or because such advice appears useful to the culture. All the while, that elder might be violating the stereotype for very (personally) functional reasons. Meanwhile, that older adult, no longer reproducing or contributing through physical work, is still working toward the good of the group by promoting group values and attitudes.

An additional complication occurs in a fast-changing technological society where custom is less valuable. The most adaptive strategy, in this case, would be to achieve a behavioral synthesis in which sex roles change or converge.

Data Relating Successful Aging and Sex-Role Flexibility

One piece of evidence is the analysis of Rorschach responses in old age [*Ames* et al., 1954]. The 'normal' subjects' Rorschach profiles were highly individualized and did not manifest sex-role-stereotyped responses to any great degree. But the 'preseniles', and to a great extent the 'seniles', responded in a sex-stereotyped way. Longitudinal follow-ups demonstrated that as normals became seniles, their responses fell into the sex-stereotyped pattern.

A second piece of evidence is found in the *Reichard* et al. [1962] study of aging and personality. In this study 87 men between the ages of 55 and 84 were interviewed. Subjects were healthy, middle-class urbanites. After extensive testing, five patterns of adjustment were noted, ranging from mature to self-hating. The men who were best adjusted manifested both activity and passivity, with neither trait dominating. They reported genuine satisfaction from their work and wanted to maintain independence. They also accepted passivity and had an awareness of their feelings and drives. A nurturing role was acceptable, as was that of nurtured one. *Reichard* concludes that growing old may make it possible for a man to integrate formerly unacceptable feminine drives into his personality due to changing social expectations. Whatever the dynamic, lessening sex-role differentiation was related to more successful aging.

Another study of personality and aging reported by *Williams and Wirth* [1965] focused on major life-styles of the successfully aging. The characteristics deemed most important to successful aging in *either* women or men were autonomy and persistence (versus precariousness or instability) in both work and family relations. Both sexes were represented by individuals who were successful in old age and who demonstrated active, independent orientations while not neglecting nurturant activities.

In testing middle-aged and old men and women with the Thematic Apperception Test (TAT), *Neugarten and Gutmann* [1968] analyzed the perceptions each age and sex group held of traits shown by old men or women in general. This study and others [*Neugarten,* 1968] pointed out that older men are expected to be more receptive to affiliative and nurturant impulses as they age, while older women are expected to be more accepting of egocentric and aggressive impulses as they age. To some degree, we see an androgynous sex-role *ideal* which is accepted by many age groups.

When *Neugarten* et al. [1964] classified old men and women into personality types and then related types to life satisfaction, integrated men and women were the most satisfied. Integrated men and women combined aggressive and passive-dependent drives, had insight into themselves and their feelings and impulses, and accepted both family and work roles.

Other studies, for example *Britton and Britton* [1972] and *Jacobson* [1974], have obtained similar indications of lessening sex-role differentiation in old age. Finally, *Jewett's* [1973] study should be mentioned. He investigated the personality traits of especially long-lived individuals. Their longevity was related to the ability to combine independence, interest in work, activity, and strength with adaptability, nurturance, family concerns, and acceptance of emotions.

Interpretation of the Studies

In spite of some flaws, the studies cited above have been generally accepted as valid by students of aging. The question of cause and effect in studies of personality and longevity is a difficult one. The only statement that can logically be made is that survival and satisfaction in old age are often *concomitant* with adoption of sex roles which combine traits culturally defined as masculine and traits culturally defined as feminine. Perhaps long-lived individuals and those satisfied in old age have always been nonconformist in this respect. Perhaps their sex roles have been modified due to recently changed situational demands such as children leaving home, retirement, or age status expectations. Malleability in such basic roles argues that sex roles are, for the most part, learned, and perhaps less central to identity than was expected by earlier theory.

Which of the possible explanations for the association between sex-role flexibility and successful aging received the most support? The first general approach, i.e. that the 'fittest' survive and role flexibility equals fitness, seems to be supported. 'Survival' can be conceptualized either as longer life, or as a better quality of life. There is evidence in all the studies cited to support the position that sex-role-flexible persons live longer and age more successfully. However, the first approach does little to elucidate the dynamic behind the association.

The second general approach was that the creative, flexible person survives, and that sex-role flexibility is but one form of creativity. There is evidence in the Jewett study that creative older adults also demonstrate sex-role flexibility. The profiles of integrated, peak-living, self-actualizing individuals described by *Maslow* [1964] include a generalized creativity. However, aging, longevity, and sex-role flexibility were not examined specifically in these studies. *Barron's* [1968] and *Arieti's* [1976] studies of the creative personality also point to a generalized flexibility and heterogeneity of interests and behaviors in this group. Again, sex-role flexibility is not specifically mentioned and investigated by *Barron* or *Arieti,* or by the authors they cite. In the area of cognition and behavioral flexibility, *Butler* [1973] notes that general flexibility correlates with lack of impairment in old age. It can be hypothesized that the survival value of sex-role flexibility is somehow tied to general creativity and flexibility, a further step toward an understanding of the association between sex-role flexibility and successful old age.

The third possible explanation for the relationship was a more detailed derivation of the second and the first. Biological, psychological, and cultural tasks *conflict* for most older adults; this conflict is apparent in the area of sex roles; the older adult who can arrive at a better synthesis of the conflicting roles and behaviors is creative and flexible and is rewarded by a more successful old age and a longer life expectancy. Evidence for the multidomain conflict surrounding sex-role behaviors and for the covariance of sex-role flexibility and successful aging was described in the studies cited above. This potential explanation goes furthest in detailing a dynamic underlying this and other adaptive behaviors, and is easiest to operationalize and test.

Riegel [1976] has described the thesis-antithesis-synthesis model which underlies this third explanation. He has also [*Riegel,* 1975] shown how the dissonance between the biological, psychological, cultural, and environmental demands on a person can lead to adult conflict and possibly to growth. Other existing theories of life span personality development [*Looft,* 1973] have been unable to incorporate so many varied aspects of adult life in this coherent way. In terms of this model, the older person's biological needs would most likely be congruent with equivalent male/female roles, and psychological needs with disparate male/female roles. Cultural needs would be congruent with disparate male/female roles (in a slowly changing traditional culture) or with equivalent roles (in a culture moving toward androgyny as an ideal). To reach a complex role which synthesizes these needs and responses and situational expectations can be a difficult growth experience, associated (direction of causality unknown) with successful aging and longevity when it does lead to growth.

Many views of development in older adults implicitly use this model. When *Erikson* [1963] speaks of crisis resolution leading to development, he appears to be describing a similar model. *Clayton* [1975] interprets *Erikson's* 'crisis' as compromise, precisely what is involved in obtaining one type of synthesis. The older individual must successfully combine the activities and demands of a lifetime into a congruent whole.

In the area of life-span sex-role development, *Hefner* et al. [1975] speak of three stages which appear to utilize this model of thesis-antithesis-synthesis: global roles; polarized roles; and transcendent roles. These authors, however, do not look at sex-role development from all three functional points of view (biological, psychological, cultural) as we have done. Even less dialectical is *Bem's* [1974] model of androgynous behavior. It may prove worthwhile to examine *Riegel's* [1975] model for its utility in examining adult growth *and* adult sex-role development.

Successful achievement of synthesis in either or both may predict successful aging and longevity.

The relationship between androgyny and successful aging appears to be part of a larger pattern of increasing and decreasing sex-role differentiation at points in the life span. At birth, the individual behaves androgynously. Sex roles diverge in middle childhood, converge again in the working period of the early 20s, and diverge again during the child-raising period. When the children have grown, roles again converge. This changing lifetime pattern suggests that sex roles are not central to identity and that the adaptive individual usually functions with the ability to modify sex roles and other roles when needed. *Block* [1973] notes that the most complex stages of *Kohlberg's* model of moral reasoning, and of *Loevinger's* model of ego development, among others, delineate behavior that can be characterized as androgynous. She suggests that the individual's integration of sex-role behaviors represents a more advanced level of development. Older adults' behavior helps confirm her point of view.

Why might behavior demonstrating sex-role flexibility lead to a more successful, long life span? Probably, it meets the biological needs of the individual, provides for psychological continuity, and does not antagonize the dominant culture. The normal, healthy (adaptive) old person, manifesting a combined male/female role, is most likely an individual who has incorporated *all* the major values of his or her culture. On the other hand, the presenile or nonadaptive old person, manifesting stereotyped masculinity/femininity like that of early childhood, appears to be less flexible, more rigid, and focused on atypical values and behaviors in the culture.

Need for Directed Studies

Although we do not know the genesis of the apparent merging of sex roles with age, we have seen some evidence that it does occur and that it does relate to successful aging. The need to study masculinity and femininity, life-span identity, and the dialectical processes is clear.

Examination of the behaviors of *unsuccessful* aging in the studies cited above tends to confirm that divergent sex roles in old age relate to less successful aging. Many questions arise. To what extent do counselors, clinicians, social workers, and others consider nonstereotyped sex-role behavior deviant in older adults? What effect does this role convergence have on the generally accepted definitions of masculinity and femininity? How integral are sex roles to life-span identity? Is there a developing androgyny for all aging cohorts? Further directed research will answer these questions.

In this chapter we examined three newer approaches to the understanding of sex roles: a cognitive, postformal approach; a general systems theory approach; and a dialectical approach. All are useful in highlighting purposes and mechanisms of sex-role development throughout the life span. When we examine sex roles in the context of cognitive functioning or in the contexts of sociobiological approaches or of history, we notice that roles seem to be components of systems that operate in almost organic ways. Like the living systems of *Miller* [1978], these systems use roles to make contact between individuals and larger systems, and to spur change or meet crises for adaptation purposes. Examining sex roles in context raises questions about the narrow ways they are typically conceptualized and suggests new research approaches that are broader in scope. In the next chapter these issues will be examined more carefully from the perspective of adaptation and species survival.

3. Adaptation Across the Life Span: Evolution, Future Shock, and Sex Roles

Our capacity to adapt successfully to social change across the life span and especially in old age depends upon a complex interaction of biological and environmental factors. In part our functioning is based on evolutionarily derived biological capacities. But these biological factors do not determine behavioral patterns in the manner of instinct but in more subtle and complex ways. Ultimately it is culture and not genetics that plays the major role in adaptation. But this is not to say that only culture is worth studying in order to fully appreciate the nature of the human adaptation process.

In this chapter the nature of the biological-environmental interaction is examined in terms of human adaptation to rapid social change. This is the kind of change which, when adaptation fails to occur, will result in what *Toffler* [1970] calls future shock. The different ways in which males and females have been socialized has resulted in a differential emphasis on certain traits for each gender. These culturally derived traits may indeed have differential adaptation capacities from a life-span perspective and particularly in old age. Traits which characterize the female gender in our culture and traits which characterize the male gender will be referred to as 'female traits' and 'male traits' in this chapter. This is not to imply that these traits have only a biological basis or that these traits characterize all males and females, but only that these are the traits chosen by Western culture as being gender-appropriate at this point in time.

Adaptation is the process by which living organisms alter their response patterns in relation to changes in the surrounding environment. The world around us changes constantly. We are required to adjust our behavior to the realities of the environment around us in order to survive, both physically and psychologically. The focus in biology is often on form, whereas psychologists tend to emphasize function and interrelationships. The underlying unity to the study of human development derives from the factor of ongoing change in the environment and the process by which we adjust to constant alterations in our surroundings. The core process of life itself is adaptation. By studying adaptation we are able to follow human development in all its aspects: biological, psychological, sociological, anthropological, and even philosophical.

Environmental stimuli affect us differently depending upon our individual adaptation levels [*Helson,* 1964]. The adaptation level for any given human being arises from the aggregate past experiences of various stimulation levels measured against current environmental stimulation. If a person experiences stimulation at a customary level to which that individual has become adapted, no adaptive response will be needed. It is only when the level of stimulation in the environment exceeds what the individual is used to that the process of adjustment which psychologists call adaptation is needed. Unfortunately, given the rate of change in the latter part of the 20th century, most people are continuously forced to adapt to stimuli beyond their comfortable, familiar adaptation levels and therefore are susceptible to the experience of future shock.

For *Homo sapiens* adaptation has special implications because among all the animals of the earth humans have the longest period of childhood and therefore of dependency on other members of their species. Thus, the relationship between dependence and independence takes on special meaning within the context of human development. Adaptation is not limited to individuals but occurs in groups as well. Culture is our greatest species adaptation. Each human culture has produced ways of dealing with the dependence/independence aspect of survival. None of us can successfully adapt to the environmental realities around us as isolate individuals. We are all affected by group norms for behavior and by the social institutions within which we must operate. Our dependency needs can only be met by other humans and our desire for independence can only develop into personal freedom with the support of others. Essentially, the human condition is one of interdependence and this comprises a large part of our adaptation capacity. The human life span covers the progression from complete dependence in infancy, to the beginnings of independence in the autonomy of the toddler to the ever increasing independence of the pre-schooler, the middle years child (6–10), the pre-adolescent, and finally the open clash between dependence and independence which characterizes adolescence. Life-span development continues with the independence of the young adult followed by the meeting of dependency needs of others as we progress further into adulthood. One of the most difficult aspects of reaching the aging part of the life span is the specter of dependence on others which is raised by declining health or economic resources. This is a major issue which must be addressed by any culture in which concern for human well-being is a priority.

Evolution, Instinct, and Sex Differences in Behavior

Evolution includes long-term, gradual, genetic changes that reflect the effects of selection pressure on species of animals in their adaptation to their environments. Instinct refers to (1) unlearned, highly stereotyped sequences of responses which result from a particular complex of stimuli; (2) a collection of physiological mechanisms which mediate the behavioral differences brought about by evolution; (3) genetically determined behaviors, and (4) complex, rigidly patterned unlearned behavior which is universal among all members of a species (of the same age and the same sex).

Learning is defined as a more or less permanent change in behavior potentiality which occurs as a result of reinforced practice, imitation, or observation. Sex differences in behavior are statistically significant differences between the average score (one standard deviation above and below the mean) for a group of females and a group of males.

Instinct and learning represent opposite strategies in the evolutionary struggle for survival. Instinct insures that reproduction of the species is a fairly automatic process. An animal is not required to learn how to attract a member of the other sex, how to mate, how to build a shelter or nesting site, and how to care for the young. All these reproductive behaviors are controlled by genetically fixed neural circuits evolved over thousands of generations within a species. Instinct produces fixed behavior patterns which are not readily modifiable. Specific stimuli trigger these genetically programmed behavioral sequences.

The strength of the instinct strategy for survival is the assurance that reproduction of the species will occur almost automatically. The weakness of the instinct strategy for survival is that a sudden alteration of the environment in which a species has evolved may eliminate critical stimulus elements of the instinct sequence. The animal cannot change its behavior pattern in response to a quickly changing environment and therefore becomes extinct.

The learning strategy for evolutionary survival is based on constant adaptation to the environment. In a sense, instinct involves adaptation of the entire species to the environment over thousands of generations whereas learning involves adaptation to the environment within the life span of the single individual member of the species. One provides the security of fixity and the other provides flexibility.

As the phylogenetic scale is ascended, instinct decreases and learning becomes the ascendant survival strategy. Among primates learning is necessary for normal emotional responding, sexual behavior, nurturant behavior, even aggressive behavior. We cannot speak of 'maternal instinct' or 'aggressive instinct' on the level of the rhesus monkey. By the time we reach the phylogenetic level occupied by *Homo sapiens,* learning represents the human strategy for survival. *Homo sapiens* is the 'learning animal', the adaptation animal. *Homo sapiens* constantly changes clothing to adapt to temperature change, goes on to change temperature via heating or air conditioning, and even goes so far as to adapt to existence in space and on the moon by creating the ultimate adaptation, a complete life-support system.

Homo sapiens is the result of millions of years of evolution focused on behavioral adaptation and flexibility as well as an ever-increasing capacity for cognitive integration, i.e. thinking. Human gender identity should be studied in light of the enormous capacity for learning which characterizes *Homo sapiens* as a species.

Clearly human behaviors are not genetically determined, stereotypic sequences, released by stimulus triggers in the environment. Just as clearly, no behavior is purely environmentally determined. Human development consists of the ongoing process of interaction between biological and environmental influences. Perhaps the term inborn propensities [*Vale,* 1980, p. 141] would best replace the term instinct in describing the complex nature of biological-environmental interaction.

The interaction between biology and environment which characterizes human development underlies the process of adaptation. 'What the genes really determine are the reaction ranges exhibited by individuals with more or less similar genes over the entire gamut of possible environments . . . similar genes may have different effects in dissimilar environments . . .' [*Dobzhansky,* 1973, p. 8]. All traits are the result of combined genetic and environmental influences. Nothing can be traced back to pure hereditary determination. All traits emerge from the DNA code through specific environmental influences. Similarly, no human trait can be attributed solely to the power of learning. All learned behavior occurs with the biologically based sensory receptor system of the human body mediating external influences. A stimulus only exists if the nervous system of the individual has been aroused by an energy source in the environment. Something is not a stimulus because it occurs in the physical world. The word stimulus is reserved for an event in the physical world which generates energy which is transduced by the appropriate organismic receptor into neuronal energy inside the individual. The electrochemical arousal of the nervous system must occur before an organism can be stimulated by something in the environment. Adaptation to changes in the environment can occur only through the physiological pathways developed through millions of years of evolution. But, at the same time, '. . . selection for trainability and cultural receptivity has been going on not in some populations and races but in the whole human species, and uninterruptedly ever since the inception of humanity and of its dependence on culture as a method of adaptation to and control of the environment' [*Dobzhansky*, 1973, pp. 93–94].

Development is the process of continual interaction between environmental and hereditary forces in the life of the human organism from conception to senescence and death. The influence of the environment is far more complex than is usually recognized. The full impact of nutrition, stimulation, disease, cultural, and psychological factors in the development of the organism must be appreciated before the nature of the environmental-genetic interaction basis to human development can fully be understood. Similarly, the limitations and capacities contained within our biological heritage (including those 'innate propensities') cannot be appreciated unless the evolutionary history which produced the biological entity which is *Homo sapiens* can be understood.

Agency and Communion in Human Adaptation

Bakan [1966, pp. 14–15] describes human existence in terms of a basic duality between agency and communion.

I have adopted the terms 'agency' and 'communion' to characterize two fundamental modalities in the existence of living forms, agency for the existence of an organism as an individual, and communion for the participation of the individual in some larger organism of which the individual is a part. Agency manifests itself in self-protection, self-assertion, and self-expansion; communion manifests itself in the sense of being at one with other organisms. Agency manifests itself in isolation, alienation, and aloneness; communion in contact, openness, and union. Agency manifests itself in the urge to master; communion in non-contractual cooperation.

Bakan [1966, p. 14] indicates that most cultures have split the agency-communion dimension along sex lines with the masculine agentic traits being valued more highly than the female communal traits. This extreme split places society in peril. 'The villain is unmitigated agency. The moral imperative is to mitigate agency with communion.'

Communal traits were the key evolutionary and survival traits in the transition from pongid (ancestral ape) to hominid and during hominid evolution. Early *Homo sapiens* was primarily communal in orientation with gatherer-hunters sharing food, cooperating, and being mutually supportive. The transition from gatherer-hunter/horticulturists to agriculturists 10,000 years ago began the transition away from communal values and towards agentic ones. *Sanday* [1981] explains this transition as stemming from the relationship of people to the physical requirements of food acquisition in a given environment. Harsh environments give rise to male creation myths, patriarchy, and sharp sex-role distinctions. The role of women in nature is degraded in these cultures and the stage is set for the ascendency of 'male' traits over 'female' traits.

Successful Aging: Androgyny or Female Sex-Role Traits?

Recent longitudinal studies have shown a relationship between successful aging and sex-role flexibility which has been characterized as androgynous [*Sinnott,* 1982]. Another aspect of successful aging may well stem from the ascendency of 'female' attributes in aging humans. These 'female' attributes originate from hominid evolution [*Tanner,* 1981], ecological patterns [*Merchant,* 1982], culture [*Bakan,* 1966], and psychological factors [*Gilligan,* 1982].

Tanner [1981, p. 11] maintains that the transition from pongids to hominids occurred because of traits developing in the females. 'The hypothesis, in brief, is that transitional hominid mothers were beginning to gather and share plants with offspring and that this female tool-use, gathering, carrying, and mother-child food-sharing became essential for the transitional population's adaptation to the new environment of the savannah.'

The trait system which has developed in women as a combination of evolution and cultural history concerns communion [*Bakan,* 1966] and morality [*Gilligan,* 1982]. With regard to moral-ethical considerations 'male and female voices typically speak of the importance of different truths, the former of the role of separation as it defines and empowers the self, the latter of the ongoing process of attachment that creates and sustains the human community' [*Gilligan,* 1982, p. 156].

Successful aging may well depend upon the ascendency of 'female' attributes in older humans: communion over agency, attachment over isolation, intimacy over nondisclosure [*Lewis,* 1978], and sensitivity to the environment [*Merchant,* 1982] over exploitation and devastation of the environment. After all, hominid evolution can be seen as particularly relevant to the beginning and end of the life span [*Petersen,* 1980], where hormonal influence is minimal and dependence is maximal. The family is much more important at the beginning and end of the life span. At the beginning of the life span the female traits which guided hominid evolution (nurturance and food gathering, sharing, and cooperation) provide for the survival of the young. At the end of the life span those same traits serve to nurture self, partners, and friends.

For women, 'identity is defined in a context of relationship and judged by a standard of responsibility and care' [*Gilligan,* 1982, p. 156]. Morality arises out of the experience of connection (communion) and is not seen as a matter of objective evaluation of claims (agency). For women morality is an outgrowth of human attachment.

The sex-role socialization system in 20th century Western culture has placed the communal sphere of human existence almost exclusively upon women. This has given rise to attributes which now differentiate women's moral judgements from men's, women's values and concerns from men's, women's emotional patterns from men's, and so on. The problem is that men are still viewed as the norm in modern society; therefore, it is always women's morality, values, concerns, and emotional expressivity which are seen as abnormal and less desirable than men's agentic qualities.

Being human involves a combination of unique *Homo sapiens* traits built onto a basic primate structure. Our primate natures are an essential part of our biological selves. An important facet of our primate as well as our hominid heritage is the social nature of *Homo sapiens.* We are a highly social species, dependent for our very survival on the nurturance and support of others, particularly at the beginning and end of the life span.

As primates we need to enhance our social interrelationships with tactile stimulation – *Harlow's* [1958] contact comfort. This is especially true in the early and late years of our lives. Female sex-role socialization in most human cultures has resulted in both the social and tactile nurturance aspects of our primate selves developing more fully in women than men. Friendship, intimacy, attachment, hugging, holding, and soothing function to sustain and enrich the lives of many older women, whereas men are more often shut off from these primate adaptation capacities by male sex-role socialization. The male sex role has been termed a health hazard [*Harrison*, 1978] which diminishes longevity in men even in the latter part of the 20th century. 'The psychosocial perspective suggests that male role expectations are limiting and unclear, turn male maturation into an achievement, and are contrary to human needs. Attempts to fulfill the role requirements result in anxiety, emotional difficulty, a sense of failure, compensatory behavior which is potentially dangerous and destructive, and stress which results in physical and premature death' [*Harrison*, 1978, p. 70].

Human learning capacity provides us with a basis for ongoing adaptation to the environment which is almost limitless. However, our emotional and psychological needs constrain the adaptive range within which our learning ability can operate. This is what leads to problems in adjustment such as *Toffler's* [1970] future shock, i.e. failure to adapt when too many changes occur around us, and the rate of change in our environment is exceedingly rapid.

The other ways in which we are unique affect and direct our adaptive capacities. *Homo sapiens* is the only species which must cope with its own mortality; we are the only animal that knows of death as personal fate. The two strategies which have emerged to deal with mortality and provide meaning to activities across the life span have been agency and communion [*Bakan*, 1966]. Agency provides an immortality of personal achievement, a legacy of accomplishments that indicate the existence of the individual. Communion establishes meaning in the universe through daily interaction with others, a social bond of support and sustenance against the futility of death. For older adults, communion becomes increasingly important as a basis for adaptation to changing environmental circumstances. Unfortunately, for the average man a lifetime of agentic orientations leaves little knowledge of communal resources for survival. This may well be a significant factor in the differential longevity of women over men.

Homo sapiens is the only animal able to choose how to live; all other animals just exist in the present. Because of our unique appreciation of the future we can live in three dimensions simultaneously: the memories of our past, the impression of the present, and the anticipation of future events. This means that we alone, among all the species, can make choices based on past learning experiences, present conditions, and anticipation of future possibilities. Choosing agentic over communal values has been a development in Western cultures; Eastern cultures tend to value communal traits. Most men have always responded to the success life-style because of the agentic quality of male sex-role socialization. Today women who wish to be successful are having agentic traits urged upon them. Yet it can be argued that the survival of Western culture itself depends upon the mitigation of agency by communion [*Bakan,* 1966].

If we choose agency over communion we are limiting the kinds of adaptive skills with which we shall deal with our own old age. By choosing agency over communion we are raising the specter of loneliness, isolation, emotional sterility, and in all likelihood a life span truncated by the effects of excessive stress. Western culture has traditionally associated communal traits with women and undervalued both. Successful aging may well depend upon the revaluing of both throughout the life span.

Historically, women have always been associated with nature [*Merchant,* 1980]. The ecological perspective is one in which the interconnectedness of environment and organism is appreciated. Women's community embeddedness and survival concerns have given them just such an ecological orientation. Achieving a balance with nature rather than exploiting and degrading nature has been more of a female approach than a male one. Sensitivity to the environment around us and skilled attempts at achieving a balance between human and environmental concerns marks women's approach to life more than men's.

Ignoring the environment around us might create even more problems in old age. Older persons are more and more constrained by the physical environment. Older persons move more slowly, are less agile, are more sensitive to environmental insults such as pollution factors. It is much more devastating when an older person lives out of harmony with the environment since the older person is less flexible in readjusting and has little time or resources to do so. This means that older people are particularly susceptible to future shock (nonadaptation to change). Older adults often do counterproductive things biologically or psychologically in reaction to the rapid pace of change in the environment.

In many ways the attributes which women have acquired through the process of sex-role socialization in our culture serve them well in old age. Friendship, intimacy, empathy, physical contact, interrelatedness, emotional expressivity, compromise, and social sensitivity combine together to enhance the survival capacity of people who can no longer control nature by the force of their own bodies but must live within the constraints of a more limited system.

It is interesting to speculate which is more useful in adapting to environmental change and avoiding future shock, these female attributes or the flexibility associated with androgyny. I suspect that the combination of male and female socialized traits which comprises androgyny is most successful in promoting adaptation to changing environmental conditions when the traits are loaded in the female or communal direction and away from the more agentic of the male traits.

Successful adaptation to the environment becomes increasingly important with aging but the ability to adapt may depend upon already having certain traits, skills, and attributes, many of which are communal in nature. The valuing of communal traits by our culture must increase if people are to transit old age successfully. Then we can all share *Bakan's* [1966, p. 236] vision that the 'proper way of dying is from fatigue after a life of trying to mitigate agency with communion'.

Joan S. Rabin

4. What Little We've Learned so Far: Theory

A number of publications focused on theory of roles are the basis for this chapter. One part of this new work addresses the nature of masculinity and femininity as constructs. A second is focused on the influence of situational factors on roles and the relation between roles and well-being. The third focus is the nature of roles in relation to self-concept, and models of change (role change) over time (the life span).

This chapter will concentrate on new work with theoretical implications for life-span sex-role research. Publications with life-span theoretical implications are reported even if they were based on research with young respondents. It should be noted that this chapter will not be an attempt to completely summarize literature on the concepts of masculinity, femininity, androgyny, or their correlates. That literature is vast, easily accessible, and largely related to younger adults. Considerations concerning measurement issues also have been omitted from this chapter, but can be found in chapter 10.

The Nature of Masculinity and Femininity

Bernard [1980] was concerned with the relationship between the dimensions measured by the BSRI and other personality dimensions. He investigated this question in both primary and replication samples of young adults by testing with the BSRI and the Sixteen Personality Factor Questionnaire. Regression analysis led to the conclusion that the masculine scale was convergent with personality dimensions characterized as masculine, but that results for the feminine scale were equivocal. Discriminant analysis demonstrated that masculine and androgynous types were different in personality characteristics from feminine and undifferentiated types. Construct validation of androgyny theory and the

BSRI was also provided by *Senneker and Hendrick* [1983] in terms of helping behavior.

Results suggested that masculinity and femininity, as traits, may be different. Femininity may be expressed under conditions of environmental salience but not under paper and pencil conditions. Self-endorsement of masculine items also may really measure 'proneness to enter a role'. Endorsement of masculine items may be perceived as rewarding since masculinity is valued by our culture.

Results of this study would reconcile the findings [*Kelly and Worell*, 1977] that the androgynous were behaviorally flexible and more adaptive with those paper and pencil results of others that the masculine adapted better. The manner in which roles influence adaptivity and the conditions under which this occurs are beginning to be investigated. Low tolerance for ambiguity has been found to mediate social competence only in androgynous females [*Heilbrun*, 1978]. This happened by means of high facial affect decoding skill and high social cognition that would allow decoded information to be used for social action. Results of this study demonstrated that studies of optimum functioning, adaptivity, and roles need to take into account the setting, the social valuation of the role behavior, the consequences of adopting the role behavior, and whether the behavior is filling out a paper and pencil survey or acting in other ways.

Joint contributions of masculinity and femininity were not uniform on the Personal Attributes Questionnaire [*Spence and Helmreich*, 1979 a, b]. Therefore, the methods of analysis using absolute scores, as opposed to scoring masculinity and femininity relative to each other, were most useful. This implies that mode of scoring must be considered in all studies.

Apparently the undesirable characteristics of several femininity-scale BSRI items were what was making that scale less related to adaptivity or adjustment [*Silvern and Ryan*, 1979]. Using an alternative scoring system with desirable femininity-scale items, the relationship between adjustment and sex-role status was altered, i.e. balanced. Superior adjustment (self-rated) was still related to androgynous roles for women but not for men, possibly reflecting the value of being masculine in the current social context.

In another study, the femininity scale of the BSRI, composed of expressive items, appeared applicable to both sexes, but the masculinity scale was not [*Petersen*, 1981]. Instrumentality, at least as measured by the short form of the BSRI, may be qualitatively different for males and females. A female or a male may be instrumental, but not necessarily in a masculine way.

Influence of Situational Factors

Locksley and Colten [1979] addressed problematic assumptions in sex-role theories of androgyny. The first issue was centered on the appropriateness of stereotype-anchored scales for assessing self-concept dimensions. The authors pointed out that stereotypical traits may be useful only in socially contrastive situations, and may not mean much personally to individuals in daily, more nebulous circumstances. They pointed out that conceptual structures for traits differ from conceptual structures for persons. The latter contain individualized information. Specific individual features may, of course, activate a part of the trait concept and cause it to be applied as a whole to that person. Any individual may be a good or a poor exemplar of a trait. The main criticism revolves around labeling as androgynous one who is so only in relation to global stereotypes and who, as an individual, may be so only some of the time in certain situations.

A second criticism was linking roles, specifically androgyny, to mental health. The authors argued that androgyny implies a freedom from what this society demands, namely freedom from more stereotyped role-related responses. But sex plays a role in the very structure of experience in this society. The adaptivity of an action depends on the situation, and in some situations which are structural in respect to sex the most adaptive act is a sex-role stereotyped one. So studies need to take into account the situational demands, the social implications of any role-related behavior, and the awareness of the actor concerning demands, effects, and choices available. Androgyny may involve the awareness of choice in known situations where the social implications of stereotyped and non-stereotyped choices are known and the actor has masculine and feminine behaviors available in his or her behavioral repertoire. This problem is addressed by *Helmreich* et al. [1979] also.

A model presented by *Worell* [1981] was used to hypothesize, in a similar vein, that the relationship between well-being and androgyny can only be expected to be positive within certain developmental periods. *Worell* further hypothesized that situational outcomes would sometimes be negative for those who chose nontraditional (androgynous) behaviors and were punished, especially if peer support was lacking. She proposed further study with a structure focusing on job assignment, job description, job satisfaction, and job performance. In support of *Worell's* theoretical position, *DeGregorio and Carver* [1980] found that adjustment was a function of comfortable fit among behavior patterns, sex-role orientation, and situational demands. These issues were also discussed by *Lenny* [1979 a, b] and *McGee and Wells* [1982], who reach similar conclusions.

Self-descriptions on the BSRI were not stable across social roles of parent, student, or boyfriend/girlfriend [*Uleman and Weston,* 1984]. When respondents described themselves across roles their answers changed significantly in 75% of the cases. *Uleman and Weston* concluded that sex-segregated social roles call for a variety of personality traits and may not be related to global sex-role stereotypes. They may instead depend on situational demands.

The hypothesis that androgyny was related to well-being was tested by *Taylor and Hall* [1982]. They also tested an alternative hypothesis that masculinity was best for males and femininity best for females. This was done by using a two-way analysis of variance model and examining the interaction term to assess androgyny. This approach directly examined the interaction rather than only the additive effects of masculinity and femininity. The most important advance was the reconceptualization of the model, but results also suggested that masculinity was associated with adaptivity, contrary to both hypotheses of *Taylor and Hall* [1982]. *Whitley* [1981] reached similar conclusions, finding that both masculinity and femininity were related to self-esteem, but masculinity was most important. But self-esteem was positively related to desirable characteristics so that the balance of traits turned out to be important. Self-esteem measures and sex-role measures often seemed to be measuring the same constructs, or certain dimensions of the same constructs. The sex-role measures also were seen to be tapping just one aspect of sex roles, a psychological one. *Whitley* suggested that the level of analysis (psychological, sociological, anthropological) must be specified. Hypotheses about centrality of sex role to one's self-concept and ideal versus real sex-role concepts might be tested. These issues were also discussed by *Lenney* [1979 a, b]. Similar results were found by *Antill and Cunningham* [1979], but results of *Whitley* [1981] using path analyses were not supportive.

Self-Concept

Self-concept, especially its development in later life, was important to *Breytspraak* [1984]. She suggested that males and females base their self-concept on different factors throughout the life span. These factors are often sex-role-related, for example, achievement and interpersonal comfort. Females' self-concepts, therefore, were more likely to be influenced by current circumstances, while males' self-concepts were not; interpersonal relations are more volatile than achievement. *Breytspraak* made the point that the self – of which sex roles are a part – can be seen in several ways, depending on one's theoretical orientation. In psychoanalytic and egoanalytic theory the self represents a conscious integration of inborn instincts and social demands. The self did not create itself apart from relations with others, or apart from an increasing awareness of its own internal desires. In humanistic psychology the self is actively striving to become all that is possible for it to be in the context of others. For experimental social psychologists the self is created in reaction to outside forces or as a concept to describe a controllable center of causality capable of action on the environment. Symbolic interactionists look upon self and society as inextricably bound, mutual creators of each other. Self is the term for that interaction. Individual interpretations of the reality 'out there' (which, in turn, is a construct of all members of society) are important, and the creator of those is the interactive self. In role theory the self is the sense of identity that comes from playing all one's social roles and extending them to new situations. Hypotheses about sex roles and their development which might be derived from these varied ideas of self would themselves be quite varied. In life-span terms, one might speculate that, in the humanistic position, the self would grow beyond roles due to actualization. A symbolic interactionist might predict a continuing evolution of the meaning of roles due to recreation of concepts of self. A role theorist might predict that roles would become more flexible due to increasing generalization to more situations over time.

The reader will notice that research questions are a function of theoretical stance, and that some stances are more popular than others. *Braden* [1982] provided an interesting examination of sex-role development with an atypical humanistic flavor. He asked professional and nonprofessional women and professional men, all middle-aged, about current aspirations and dreams for the future. The groups differed in current reports along expectable sex-role-related lines. But when dreams for the future were analyzed all group and gender differences disappeared. Roles were associated with current life, but not with the hoped-for, fully actualized self individuals intended to become.

Sex-role theory was related to cognitive theories of sex-role identity to raise questions about psychological constructs underlying measures of sex-role attributes [*Storms*, 1979]. *Kagan* theorized that individuals compare their attributes to stereotypes to arrive at a relativistic self-concept of sex-role identity; *Kohlberg* [1966] suggested that individuals use an early established concept of themselves as masculine or feminine to mediate effects of stereotypes on developing attributes. Data supported *Kohlberg's* model. This implied that attributes and stereotypes, while correlated with each other and related to identity, may not be expressing all of the complex identity in the initial self-concept. This also implied that the expression of the self-concept could change over time as self-concept or stereotypes change over time. The cognitive approach further implied that stereotypes are schema abstracted from the environment by the knower, and therefore are far from clear or absolute. For a theoretical controversy similar in flavor to this one, the reader may wish to see *Bem* [1981a, 1982], *Crane and Markus* [1982] and *Mills and Tyrrell* [1983] on gender schema versus self-schema approaches to sex-role development. Along these same lines, *Andersen and Bem* [1981] made a cogent argument that sex-typed individuals have a particular readiness to encode and organize information in terms of gender.

The theoretical position that roles present ways of dealing with the demands of a social or life-stage situation was explored as part of *Weg's* [1983] discussion of sexuality in later years. In that volume, *Datan and Rodeheaver* [1983] discussed the changes in the nature of human loving over the life span. While old stereotypes of roles may linger, desires and demands change. The woman once chosen for her sexual restraint and nurturance is now desired for her active sexual participation with her spouse. The man chosen for his aggressive style is now asked to become intimate and expressive. Learning to love over time seemed to demand unlearning early role stereotypes and behaviors. The authors suggested that the change is from a focus on goals, e.g. generativity in love, to a focus on present experience (the 'now'). If this is so, then sexuality in later years demands a way of being, devalued in Western culture but accepted in Eastern thought and most clearly aligned, in sex-role terms, with femininity. Increasing femininity (by a broader definition), all things being equal, should then relate to better loving relationships in midlife and beyond, and should be associated with higher self-esteem in the interpersonal area. *Livson* [1983], in the same volume, suggested that androgynous personalities might be expected to be conflicted in early adulthood but less so later, with men and women taking different paths to reach that nonconflicted state.

Males and females have differing patterns of decision-making [*Moreland* et al., 1979]. Sex roles were related to use of intuitive and rational decision-making styles for females, but sex roles were related to use of only rational decision-making style for males. Females apparently could view themselves as both feminine and masculine in type (or androgynous) and endorse either decision style. But any males who included a component of femininity did not endorse a rational style. Results were interpreted to indicate that, for the females, sex-role expansion was occurring. They were adding a masculine component to the already present feminine one. Conclusions related to males were not clear.

Three models of change might be useful to consider in explorations of sex-role development over time [*Bernard,* 1976]. Change may come by increments, innovations, or diffusion; change might come by elimination of some suddenly nonadaptive approach; or change might come when a state of readiness is reached so that one more small shift leads to a large qualitative difference overall. Change might therefore be dependent on past levels of some trait, or might depend on current levels of it, or might depend on the rate of previous shifts. Change might include elements of role redefinition by society, leading to intrinsic role conflicts. A discussion of male sex-role definitions, problems, and sources of change which gives an example of these issues is found in *Pleck* [1976]. *Lenney* [1979 a, b] offered a model for sex-role development which might take individual change into account. Individuals' sex-role behavior depended, in this model, upon global self-description as masculine, feminine, or androgynous and upon their cognitive (belief system), affective (anxiety, emotional responsiveness), and motivational (goals and ideal images) orientations. A more phenomenological approach to life-span role development is also called for by *McGee and Wells* [1982], who suggested that a respondent's own view of the situation and role be incorporated into any analysis.

In summary, recent theoretical work has demonstrated the complexities of reaching a meaningful measurement of masculinity, femininity, androgyny, adjustment, or self-concept. Few investigators can hope to address all the issues raised above, but more can be conscious of them in interpreting data. Together, all of the authors seemed to be urging use of a complex model for change and for any role-related behavior. The perceptions of the respondent – about the meaning of items, about social sanctions, about situational salience – stand out as factors to be attended to in future work as soon as means can be found to measure them. Researchers considered: the nature of adaptivity in a social setting; social approval and disapproval of role-related behaviors; the utility of stereotype-based scales, especially in predicting everyday behavior; developmental stage needs; social-cognitive aspects; theoretical approaches; and idiographic considerations. All these topics led to greater awareness of the difficulty of knowing a social reality which is co-constructed by all participants and changing over time. The biological, the cognitive, the identity, the social, and the historical aspects of the situation must be addressed in sex-role development research.

5. Recent Empirical Studies:
Ten Important Conclusions

Within the last 5 years a number of reports were published on the topic of sex roles and aging. Other recent reports have dealt with sex-role theory, although they were not always written with a life-span perspective. In this chapter are described recent empirical studies with older subjects. About a third of the recent work focused on older adults, at least in part.

Recent research has built upon new trends in conceptualizing sex roles and upon the new interest in sex roles in later life. Developmental models imply that age-related changes in role might be expected as a part of normal development in mature years. Social-learning models imply that older adults learn to be less traditionally masculine or feminine as time goes by and such traditional behaviors are less likely to be reinforced.

Androgyny

There is some evidence that elders can be expected to score 'androgynous'. *Foley and Murphy* [1977] tested sex-role attributes of older males and females and found that as cohort age increased, each sex incorporated characteristics of the other while retaining sex-appropriate characteristics. In effect, they became androgynous in *Bem's* terms. The ideal selves reported included even more characteristics of the opposite sex than descriptions of actual characteristics.

In a study of adults at four transition points in life [*Lowenthal* et al., 1975], sex-role behaviors did not converge conceptually in old age. The changes that occurred appeared to be in expressive behavior: older men expressed more tenderness, or more dependency, while older women expressed more autonomy or more dominance [*Turner,* 1977].

Research has addressed the potential for sex-role-related traits to contribute to the organization of personality. *Costa and McCrae* [1977] analyzed cross-sectional differences in masculinity and femininity for adult men. Sex role was conceptualized as a bipolar trait. The Strong Vocational Interest Blank and the Cattell 16PF were among the schedules administered to people aged 25–82. The results indicated that the masculinity/femininity dimension in personality becomes a less powerful organizing variable as life progresses. In young adults, it functions to order a wide set of interests, traits, and abilities. With increasing age, the contrast between masculine and feminine attributes is less distinct, and the dimension is less valuable for ordering.

Hubbard et al. [1979] asked middle-aged and older respondents to compare themselves and their mates now and when they were first married using these categories: decision-making, advice-seeking, dependency, need for achievement, and assertiveness. Middle-aged adults' responses generally indicated personality styles that were sex-differentiated, while older adults reported changes in the direction of greater sex-role diffusion, most frequently noting spouses' motivational, retirement, and personality changes as causal factors. Thus, factors in the transition from middle to old age may lead to the appearance of androgynous behaviors as the individual adjusts to his or her own aging process.

Studies of personality in adulthood [*Neugarten,* 1964; *Neugarten and Gutmann,* 1968] provided the first indication that respondents do not describe male and female roles for older cohorts in the same way that they describe such roles for younger cohorts. *Neugarten and Gutmann* [1968] administered the TAT to men and women aged 40–70. The sample was varied in terms of social class: males were employed in both blue collar and professional occupations; females were generally housewives. The characteristics ascribed to individuals on the TAT cards varied in terms of the age and sex of the stimulus person and the age of the respondent. Younger male stimulus characters were expected to be active, involved, and aggressive, while older male stimulus characters were expected to be authoritative but submissive and passive, withdrawn from the outside world. Similarly, young female stimulus characters' attributes differed from old female stimulus characters' attributes. Younger women were thought to be deferential and undefined as personalities, while older women were described as key family figures, complex, and authoritative. By attributing such divergent characteristics to different age/sex cohorts, respondents suggested longitudinal or cohort differences in perceived normative sex roles.

The findings described above are at variance with the traditional view that females of any age are mainly passive and communal, while males of any age are mainly aggressive and agentic. *Barrows and Zuckerman* [1976] reported that males show an increase in feminine interests and attitudes with age. *Douglas and Arenberg* [1978] reported that masculinity declined in older males as measured by the Guilford-Zimmerman Temperament Survey. *Silverman* [1977] found that college students viewed 65-year-old males as significantly more feminine than 25-year-old males. In general, age or cohort trends suggest polarized sex roles are present and expected for the young, and complex combinations of femininity and masculinity are expected of and reported by the old.

Learning Roles from Life Events

Women's experiences in role discontinuity, which are inevitable as their assigned parental and spousal roles shift to postparental and widowhood roles, may teach them to be adaptive about roles and activities [*Kline,* 1975]. *Palmore* [1965] has noted that a man's work role, perceived as his greatest reinforcer, is withdrawn in old age, and this pushes him to shift from a polarized masculine role.

Age changes elicit socially desirable instrumental and expressive ('masculine' and 'feminine') attributes that take place as individuals move from adolescence to middle age and as they assume marital and adult responsibilities [*Spence and Helmrich,* 1979 a, b]. Complex life circumstances relatively unique to a given individual may cause definite changes in instrumental and expressive traits; as a result of such events, instrumentality and expressiveness may increase or decrease. Other investigators agree. *Abrahams* et al. [1978] found that sex-role concepts and sex-role attributes of both men and women change in response to changing life situations. Both sexes, when involved in situations requiring predominantly feminine behavior, described themselves as more feminine than their contemporaries who were in other situations. The same pattern of findings held for masculinity.

Several examples of this learning process have been provided by *Gutmann* [1975, 1985], who sees the distinctive sex roles of young parents as precipitated by the needs of their offspring for physical and emotional security. The father forgoes dependency needs and expressivity that might interfere with his role as main provider of physical protection. The mother, who is the primary provider of emotional security, sets aside aggressive behavior that might harm the child or alienate her spouse. As the children take over responsibility for their own security, the parents are freed to express the qualities they gave up during the time of attention to childrearing. Similar findings concerning the endorsing of distinctive sex roles by parents were reported by *Zaks* et al. [1979]. Thus, life events may impact upon the particular sex-role characteristics that a person cultivates at a given point in his or her life.

Less traditional sex roles may also emerge because of variations in family structure from the normative patterns of the past. *Livson* [1976] and *Sedney* [1977] examined life crises and transitions and their effects on sex-role development in middle-aged women. *Livson* notes that women are first socialized to marriage and family roles, but that many marriages now end in divorce. This conflict in role expectations is strongest for women in their 40s and is compounded by the traditional role restructuring that may be necessary when children leave home.

Livson [1976] followed the experiences of a group of healthy, middle-aged women from a longitudinal sample. Two different types of women were functioning successfully by age 50. One type, the 'traditionals', were conventional, sociable, and nurturing, and gained their main satisfaction from relationships. The second type, the 'independents', were intellectual and achievement-oriented, and many had successfully made the transition from divorce. Their sex-role-traditional and sex-role-independent styles were associated with their individual experiences.

Women may handle experiences differently over time. *Sedney* [1977] talked with middle-aged women between the ages of 45 and 57 about their coping responses to stressful life events. Of 80 narratives, 12 indicated that the participant reported a change in her way of handling experience over time. The majority of these cases (10 of the 11) involved the addition of 'masculine' responses to what was initially a 'feminine' set of responses.

The development or suppression of androgynous characteristics often appears to be dependent upon events in an individual's life that initiate a role shift rather than upon age itself [*Zaks* et al., 1979]. Thus, sex-role characteristics and their adaptive value at any stage of life should be related to the needs of individuals in their current life situations. In addition, findings of *Zaks* and her associates support the view that sex-role development in adulthood is profoundly affected by the timing of various life events.

Individuals undergoing stressful life events may find their traditional sex-role behaviors inadequate. The positive aspects of femininity, such as warmth and tenderness toward others, are not the most adaptive forms of response in certain situations nor are the masculine traits of independence and assertiveness always healthy responses to stress. By learning to integrate femininity and masculinity modes, individuals are better able to cope with life events in adulthood [*Turner,* 1977].

People are in constant interaction with a changing environment. The mature years involve a complex set of life periods, each with its own specific developmental potentials as well as specific events which may include risks and losses [*Gutmann* et al., 1979]. Powerful energies within the person that are no longer needed for family and job responsibilities can provide the basis for new dimensions within the personality or for certain expressions of psychopathology [*Butler and Lewis,* 1973]. Traditional adult sex roles have been associated with mental health symptomatology [*Dohrenwend and Dohrenwend,* 1969; *Gove, 1972 a, b; Manis,* 1968].

Well-Being

The findings of *Neugarten* et al. [1968] provided early evidence for the idea that the most satisfied, active elder of either sex was the individual who has integrated passive and aggressive and communal and agentic facets of the personality. More recently, *Sinnott* [1977] analyzed the evidence for adaptiveness of androgyny in old age. Based on an investigation of personality studies, clinical literature, longevity literature, and age-status expectation reports, she concluded that the typically healthy elder is both masculine and feminine in traits perceived as part of personality and in his or her view of the ideal self. This androgynous state appears to be an adaptive response to the conflicts in biological, psychological, and cultural demands upon older adults.

Sex-role identity, health behaviors, and perceived health were related in elderly females [*Skinner,* 1979]. Androgynous women rated their health good while near-feminine and feminine women rated it fair or good in a 50:50 ratio. However, near-feminine women hardly ever worried about their health while the androgynous and the feminine did. Androgynous women seldom felt their lives were useless while half the more feminine women did. *Windle* [1986, in press] categorized older adults as androgynous, masculine, feminine, or undifferentiated using the BSRI. Sex-role categorization was not predictive of either cognitive flexibility or life satisfaction.

The relationship between masculinity, femininity, and social competence in three generations of women was examined [*Gillett* et al., 1977]. The women ranged in age from 18 to 94 years. The BSRI [*Bem,* 1974] and the Texas Social Behavior Inventory [*Gillett* et al., 1977] were administered. Middle-aged women obtained higher androgyny scores than their college-age daughters and their elderly mothers. (Of course, it is possible that the results represented a cohort effect.) Because social competence was less and less related to femininity in the women as age increased, the authors hypothesized that stereotypically feminine characteristics become nonfunctional as women age. For example, during the anticipated 10 years of widowhood that most women will experience, they may need to develop competency in stereotypically masculine tasks such as financial management. They may also need to become more assertive and decisive in order to cope effectively with their environment [*Sinnott,* 1977].

It may be that the masculine attributes of an individual are more important to psychological adjustment than the presence of a balance between masculine and feminine attributes. In *Cherry and Zarit's* [1979] study of young and old women, the presence of masculine self-descriptions was related to lower reported symptoms of anxiety and depression. *Zaks* et al. [1979] found that life satisfaction correlated with masculinity in that the more subjects endorsed the masculine sex-role items, the more satisfied they were. It might also be true that the more 'masculine' subjects did not permit themselves to acknowledge symptoms and dissatisfaction.

Increased knowledge of and sensitivity to one's inner self and outward behaviors may create the ability and motivation to make changes leading to more satisfaction as one ages. However, the amount of adaptive energy reserve a person has available as he or she ages is highly individualized. It depends upon the nature, number, and intensity of biological changes, shifts in the social environment, changes in the physical surroundings, and psychological dimensions of the person's life situation [*Bell,* 1978]. *Havighurst* [1953] has described certain biosocial development tasks of later maturity as involving: (1) adjusting to decreasing physical strength and health; (2) adjusting to retirement and reduced income; (3) adjusting to death of spouse; (4) establishing an explicit affiliation with one's age group; (5) meeting social and civic obligations, and (6) establishing satisfactory physical living arrangements.

The onset of age and related life events that may have the capacity to be growth-producing in some individuals also may create mental health problems in others. *Gutmann* et al. [1979] have identified two types of psychopathology in this area. One group was composed of people who had depressive symptoms during this middle-aged period of their lives. A second group, mainly in their late 60s and 70s, was shocked by the threat of death, awareness of the life cycle, or the loss of a significant person in their lives and developed symptoms later in life.

In the first group, the men and women were threatened by the sub-merged aspects of their own personalities. For the women the depression was seen as a retreat to passivity in the face of strengths and capacities that had not been acknowledged. The women feared that acknowledge-ment of such 'masculine' qualities would mean the loss of a husband, so they exaggerated a dependent state by becoming physically and/or emotionally ill. The men who became ill in the post-parental years had shifted toward being dependent and passive in their relationships with their wives; however, the wives had moved toward autonomy and assertion and were not interested in playing an indulgent mother role to their husbands. By becoming ill, these men brought their passive needs to the hospital, the one major institution in our society that recognized and insists on a dependent stance.

The second group, mainly older women, suffered from real losses to which they had reacted catastrophically. They responded to loss of beauty as though it were a personal insult; they responded to expected losses of family and friends as though they had lost part of themselves; and they were terrified and/or enraged by the finitude of life.

Role changes that are involved within the developmental tasks not-ed above require older persons to incorporate new knowledge, alter be-havior, and thus change their definitions of themselves [*Bell,* 1978]. This is a large task that might be very stressful. Certain psychological changes must occur for androgyny to emerge [*Wells,* 1979]. The individual must integrate positive qualities of masculinity and femininity. These essen-tial psychological changes for men include: (1) a redefinition of self-confidence so that it is grounded in interpersonal sensitivity as an addition to personal power; (2) personal control that allows self-disclos-ure, and (3) valuing and enjoying both feminine and masculine behaviors [*Gross,* 1978]. The psychological changes for women can be described as

(1) the development of self-worth grounded in interpersonal as well as individual accomplishment and (2) the integration of interpersonal sensitivity with assertiveness [*Wells,* 1979].

Change over Time

The extent to which shifts in sex-role characteristics are dependent upon developmental changes separate from or interwoven with current and past life events is unclear. Sex-role characteristics also change with changing societal expectations concerning appropriate sex-role behavior. These three factors – social expectations concerning sex roles, particular current and past life events, and normal developmental changes occurring over the life span – can influence people to change their sex-role attitudes and behaviors. Evidence can be found to support the influence of all these factors. Older androgynous individuals may have experienced one or more of these factors as influential in their lives.

Recent studies of sex roles in mature and old adults addressed many topics and were therefore difficult to categorize. In these studies 'old' may have referred to a person 50 years old or to one who is 95. In some reports only older respondents were examined; in others old and young, by some definition, were compared. Most involved both females and males.

Some reports related sex roles to flexibility, self-esteem, life events, creativity, life satisfaction, health, and transactions with the environment. *Smith* [1981] investigated the impact of age on gender roles to compare older males and females on definitions of gender-role attributes, perceived masculine and feminine attributes, and the effects of subjects' environments on these attributes. Although age seemed to have some impact on changing gender roles, environment and socialization experiences had more. In environments with strong affiliative support systems, feminine gender attributes increased and masculine ones decreased for both males and females.

Few aged individuals with an androgynous sex role report significantly greater satisfaction with life than aged individuals with stereotyped sex roles [*O'Sullivan,* 1980]. For males satisfaction was not any greater; for females stereotyped were happier. Young women reported greater acceptance of masculine self-descriptions than older women. Older men reported greater acceptance of feminine self-descriptions than younger men.

Women aged 20–59 demonstrated demographic, attitudinal, time utilization, and personality differences consistent with sex typing using BSRI median splits [*Hoffman and Fidell,* 1979]. Those typed feminine rated lower in socioeconomic status (SES), education, and income, and had more homemaking and childcare responsibilities and a more conservative attitude about the role of women. Those typed masculine or androgynous had higher education, had an internal locus of control (not supported by *Hancock* [1978] for women) and higher self-esteem, and had reduced homemaking and childcare responsibilities and more liberal attitudes about the role of women. The masculine-typed group, compared with the androgynous, also had high income and SES, were less religious, and actively disliked housework. The androgynous, compared with the sex-typed, were more stable and less neurotic.

Age and sex-role expectations have been found to interact for younger and older persons [*Suzuki,* 1979]. Self-esteem scores were highly correlated with masculinity scores regardless of gender or age. Older men showed diminished endorsement of masculine characteristics. *Suzuki* concluded that sex-role identity changes with age and developmental stage for both college students and older adults.

Sex-role diffusion has been found to take place in middle-aged and older adult married couples [*Hubbard,* 1979]. Both masculine and feminine personality styles and behaviors existed in the same person, and this was more true for the older respondents. Older adult couples were also more likely to share activities assigned to one sex. Older adults also saw much more change in themselves in regard to roles than middle-aged couples did.

Women who held the most traditional attitudes about the role of women reported greater numbers of problems in old age [*Bell,* 1978]. *Bell* hypothesized that women who have been least restricted by their femaleness and have had experiences less probable for females seemed to be least limited when they assume the less desirable age category of 'old'.

Older men and women with androgynous roles sometimes report higher life-satisfaction than sex-typed peers [*Wish,* 1976]. This hypothesis was supported by correlational results but not by analysis of variance results. Young women in this sample accepted more masculine sex-role self-descriptions than the older women did. Older men were significantly more androgynous than younger men.

Murphy [1976] examined the potential discrepancy between the real and ideal self in regard to sex roles. It was hypothesized that older men would rate themselves lower in competence and higher in warmth-expressiveness than younger men, but higher in competence and equally as warm as younger women. Older males and females did not differ from each other in current sex-role identity, but older males wanted, ideally, to be more competent. Older males viewed themselves as equally competent and more warm than younger males. Older females viewed themselves as more competent but as warm as younger females. Health was related to competence. There were no differences between ideal and real self-descriptions for males or females of any age.

Beliefs about generations' behaviors did not vary as a function of generation membership. *Cameron* [1976] asked young, middle-aged, and old adults to judge which of three generations was most or least masculine or feminine in overall personality style, interests, and gender skills, and which was most or least pressured by society to do masculine or feminine sorts of things. He also asked respondents to rate themselves as to sex-role characteristics. Self-report and belief about generations did not vary as a function of membership in a generation. Young and middle-aged were believed most feminine and middle-aged the most masculine. Social pressure was seen as falling most heavily on young adults and middle-aged. The old were judged second in feminine skills and judged least along other dimensions.

Alpaugh [1975] examined the relation between sex-role identification and creativity across the adult life span in males and females. The masculinity-femininity scale of the Minnesota Multiphasic Personality Inventory (MMPI) was used. It was hypothesized that the more creative the person, the looser would be his or her sex-role identification. Degree of sex-role identification or rigidity of sex-role identification was not found to be related to creativity over the life span.

When asked to judge to what extent they had changed as a person over a 5- and a 20-year interval, young and old, male and female adults reported feeling that they had changed [*Bliwise*, 1980]. Respondents in their 40s were most likely to perceive changes, reporting that they had become more mature and interpersonally invested. Those in their 50s and 60s reported mellowing; those in their 70s and 80s reported little change.

Zaks et al. [1979] were concerned with effects of both age and life stage demands on the expression of sex role by young, middle-aged, and older respondents. They hypothesized that intimacy, parenting, grandparenting, and work would all have effects. They found that age, work status, and being a grandparent did not influence expression of a masculine, feminine, or androgynous role. Having children was associated with males and females increasing their endorsement of a feminine role. Married or never-married males were more masculine and less androgynous than separated, divorced, or widowed males. Married or never-married females were more androgynous than the remaining females.

Sex-role identity and self-esteem were related in respondents between the ages of 17 and 89 [*Puglisi and Jackson,* 1980–81]. Both males and females displayed peak masculinity scores in the middle years with no significant changes in femininity scores. Androgynous males and females displayed the highest self-esteem scores, followed by masculine, feminine, and undifferentiated, respectively. Masculinity was the best predictor of self-esteem.

To assess effects of age and cultural change in degree of sex-role stereotyping, *Urberg* [1979] studied individuals from 12 to 65 years of age. Adults were least likely to stereotype. Males and females described themselves in almost identical terms but stereotyped when describing an opposite-sex ideal person. This last result was similar to that in a study by *Eagly and Steffen* [1984] with younger respondents in which the average woman and man were perceived stereotypically when little was known about their occupation.

In summary, these studies sometimes had conflicting results but generally yielded information on a number of issues. Many investigators reported age-related shifts in role behaviors. Some reported effects on sex roles from environmental pressures. Androgynous persons frequently displayed different behaviors than sex-typed respondents, and sometimes these behaviors were very desirable ones. Masculinity was also associated with positive behaviors in some studies. These overall results suggested that developmental changes in sex roles and role-related behaviors were worthy of further investigation, and that context or environment merited attention, too. Either androgyny or masculinity or both might be optimal roles for later adulthood.

Ten Important Conclusions for Sex-Role Research

From the early and the recent literature on sex-role development and from the new approaches in chapter 2, several conclusions can be drawn. *We must not jump to conclusions that responses on a scale will be predictive of behavior.* Individuals may say that they are 'masculine' by their scale responses, but may mean they are masculine in regard to stereotyping concepts. They may rate themselves differently in other situations, act other than their ratings, and vary from situation to situation. They may do what is most rewarding and that may happen to be masculine. They may score themselves masculine due to development of an identity labeled masculine. They may do so since masculine behavior is socially desirable. They may change in self-definition due to life-stage demands, or when their own concept of masculinity is no longer like their behavior, even if to everyone else they are still 'masculine' by some other definition. And they may label themselves or act as they perceive society expects them to do. Since all these may underlie their responses to the scale, it is hard to predict behavior.

Responses to sex-role instruments do mean something. What they mean may be tempered by each person's perception of unspoken situational constraints and other factors mentioned above. If individuals respond appropriately they are matching themselves to global standards designed to reflect the most clear opposition between gender-assigned roles.

Masculinity, femininity, and androgyny have been shown to be adaptive. Depending upon the situational demands, subject to the constraints above, any of the roles might be adaptive. The real question is: What is the most useful role in a certain setting: masculine, feminine, both, or neither? Useful may mean 'liable to be rewarded' or 'consistent' or 'workable by some external criterion'. Androgyny may be the most adaptive response in terms of the last criterion; masculinity may be the most adaptive in terms of the first.

Sex roles are meaningful in terms of social expectations. The concept of global oppositional gender-linked roles is present for all members of society, and society imposes these role expectations on individuals so long as the real characteristics of those individuals are not known. So whatever complex designation of role and behavior one adopts, the general 'other' is still seen as conforming to the global stereotypes. Individuals also read role expectations projected by others and, to the degree they are conformists, attempt to conform to them.

Sex roles are meaningful ways to organize one's sense of self as socially efficacious, to create a sense of personal conformity, and to organize self-concept. The creation of the self-concept is partially accomplished by acting and noticing that the self is the center of effective acts. Roles permit structured action that is likely to work in a society. They also are labels that live beyond the individual and can be generalized to many situations. Knowing someone's sex role, without knowing the meaning of that role to the person, is to take only half a step toward knowledge.

The meaning of sex roles depends on age and developmental stage. Meanings are related to modes of cognition and social demands at each period. They are also related to the previous history and experience of the person and the historical period in which the society finds itself. Infants can know roles in direct physical forms, but cannot know them abstractly. The concrete operational person can know roles in the abstract, and the formal operational person can build logical systems of roles. The postformal person can see roles relativistically, as co-created by persons in them.

Models of sex-role changes over time can be of many types. Change can be more complex than increase or decrease in global qualities. Change might occur on one dimension but not on another, or in global role traits but not in behavior, or vice versa. Change might be triggered by specific events, or might represent an accretion over time. It may be reversible. Change might result from diffusion of a self-concept until its meaning is so muddled that it can become something new. Change might depend on past rates of change. It is useful for investigators to be clear about their underlying model of change as they discuss sex-role development.

Sex-role complexity and later-life sex-role development may be linked to cognitive abilities such as postformal thought and problem-solving skills. Roles have been linked to cognitive processes such as concept formation. As cognitive operations become more complex, their associated roles might be seen as multifaceted rather than unidimensional. They might also be seen as relativistic, i.e. conceptualizable only in relation to a certain set of beliefs or a certain situation. In adulthood a person discovers that roles do not exist 'out there' as given but instead depend partly on one's own thinking processes and moment-to-moment cognitive creations. At that point the person is thinking in a complex way that some [*Commons* et al., 1984; *Sinnott,* 1984b] would say is beyond *Piaget's* [1948] formal operations. Postformal thinkers might be more capable of androgynous concepts or sex-role transcendence.

Sex-role development questions (e.g. 'Am I being feminine?', 'What is the masculine thing to do at my age?') may be conceptualized in decision theory or problem-solving theory terms as ill-structured problems [*Wood,* 1983]. This means among other things that they have an unclear goal. Decisions must be made about the nature of the goal as a part of solving the problem. Problem-solving literature can be a guide to dimensions we need to test to understand the process of solving sex-role behavior/self-concept problems. This application of cognitive theory has not yet been attempted.

Sex-role developmental theory suggests 'new' physics concepts and might make use of them. The development of sex roles over time is the development of two interfacing systems in motion. It involves the kinds of dynamics described in relativistic and quantum physics [*Sinnott,* 1981]. From the literature reviewed it is clear that a multivariate approach needs to be taken in sex-role studies, and that adjacent centers of causality – other persons, the social order – cause changes in an individual's sex roles. The person, in turn, causes changes in the social order by his or her perception of roles, and action on that perception. It is clear that one's vantage point in measuring sex roles is very important in drawing conclusions about the results. These ideas have companion ideas in the physical sciences which could be used in studies of change in a person and among systems.

The most useful laws of life-span development may be those that apply analyses and models of the 'new' physics. This approach can take into account the conceptual distance between two or more individuals, the developmental rate of one relative to the other, and the effects of changes in other persons or events in that same interpersonal space. This may be what individuals do when they solve the problem of which sex role to identify with or to act out.

Sex-role development theory can make use of ideas in systems theory. Personal and social systems are connected by many roles, among them sex roles. Theories of living systems [*Miller,* 1978] give us an outline of the processes within and between those two systems. The flow of information can be studied within and between systems, and roles are part of that information flow. A study of system boundaries can be conceptualized as a study of rigid or flexible roles and the capability of society or a person to perceive or enact them. Future studies can take this model of living systems into account.

6. What Mature Adults Think about Sex Roles – A Study

In light of the prescriptions for sex-role research outlined at the conclusion of the preceding chapter, an investigation into the many factors in sex-role development in mature and late adulthood was carried out. That investigation is described in the next four chapters. Results and conclusions are in chapters 8 and 9, methodology in chapter 7, and, in the present chapter, the rationale and research questions for the study can be found.

The study involved interviewing 364 community-dwelling mature adults in order to determine whether they generally described themselves as androgynous or sex-typed; whether current life experiences, past life-event milestones, or perceived social expectations about roles might be related to described sex roles; and whether sex-role complexity is associated with successful aging. The results will be organized around these questions and around the hypotheses below.

The current study of sex roles and aging was undertaken from a perspective which incorporates and enlarges on previous approaches to life-span sex-role development. This perspective is both developmental and learning-oriented. This approach is developmental in that it is based on an assumption that complexity in sex-role development is a stage that presupposes earlier, less complicated stages and does not occur before these earlier stages in any individual's life span. Because the complex, androgynous stage is assumed to develop after the polarized and undifferentiated stages, older adults could be expected to display androgynous characteristics more often than young persons would. The hierarchy of stages which culminates in androgynous roles is assumed to be related to regular, age-related biological and cognitive developments. The older individual is biologically past the reproductive period and the childrearing period and need not display sex-role behavior linked to those tasks. The older person is assumed to have acquired enough complex intellectual operations to permit the understanding of a complex role. Developmentally, then, the older adult is viewed as having the capabilities to incorporate a complex sex role.

Learning is also expected to play a part in the older adult's sex role. Learning might occur in response to social expectation of a complex role; it might result from the reinforcement contingencies of the elder's current life situation; and it might result from a series of earlier life experiences which were salient enough to have a permanent impact. For some older adults all three types of learning might have occurred. Learning, then, might reinforce the developmental readiness to utilize a complex sex role, or it might run counter to such readiness. In either case, it would have an effect on sex-role characteristics.

In conceptualizing the perspective on sex-role development, it may help to imagine the case of a recently widowed older woman. Biologically she is beyond her childbearing and childrearing years, so that any traditionally masculine aspects of her personality which were not expressed because of species-serving reproductive constraints might now be freely exhibited. Cognitively she can coordinate and understand several roles at once because she has integrated the role of wife with those of daughter and friend. She perceives a general social expectation that she must now be more independent and dominant than she was as a wife. She must be in charge of her own life in addition to being feminine. She recalls that the most important milestones of her past life have involved her former job and her marriage, both involving learning and developmental aspects unique to her. She now finds herself in a situation where she will be rewarded both for obtaining a new job and for maintaining her affectional ties with her children. In her total situation, developmental and learning experiences unite in promoting an androgynous sex role. For her, such an androgynous role is more adequate than a traditional polarized feminine role or a traditional polarized masculine role in that the woman has characteristics that enable her to gain rewards from her job and from her relationship with her children. A setting less favorable toward the development of an androgynous role would be one in which the widow had children who rewarded her for dependent behavior only. Such a situation could generate conflict and a less satisfying outcome for the woman.

Figure 2 presents a diagram which describes the impact of the bio-

Fig. 2. Illustration of the theoretical perspective on sex-role identity utilized in current study: current life situation of an elderly widow

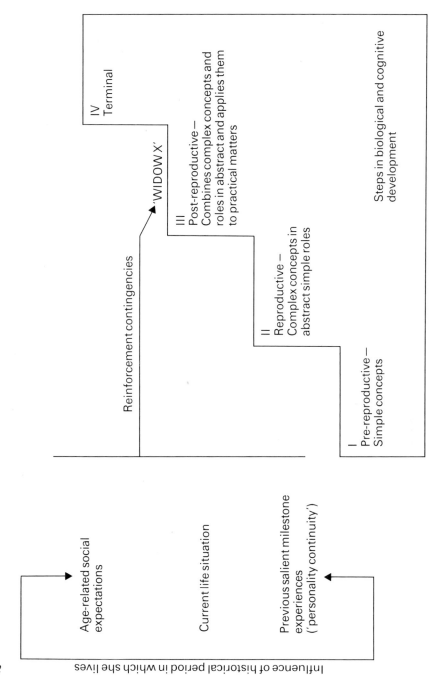

Reinforcement contingencies

'WIDOW X'

IV
Terminal

III
Post-reproductive –
Combines complex concepts and
roles in abstract and applies them
to practical matters

II
Reproductive –
Complex concepts in
abstract simple roles

I
Pre-reproductive –
Simple concepts

Steps in biological and cognitive
development

Age-related social
expectations

Current life situation

Previous salient milestone
experiences
('personality continuity')

Influence of historical period in which she lives

2

logical, psychological, social, and historical forces which may have an impact on older people. All these factors may jointly operate to influence behavior in a given situation; thus, older people must seek to understand their total situations rather than focusing only on particular forces that seem most relevant or most easily comprehended.

In the current study it was theorized that older individuals who are developmentally ready to utilize a complex role and who are reinforced for doing so will be the elders who age most successfully. If elders presented a simple sex role, the reason for such behavior was expected to be found in their assumptions of what society expected of them, or in their current life situation demands, or in their salient learning experiences over the years.

In the current study we asked which sex roles elders describe for themselves; why they describe those roles, and what difference those roles might make in their lives. The general findings were expected to follow these directions: elders describe mainly androgynous roles; roles generally fit social expectations, current life experiences, and salient milestone events, and androgynous elders age more successfully than other sex-type groups.

Specific Objectives

Primary objectives of the study were: examination of self-perceived sex roles of elders, and exploration of the relationship between complexity and type of perceived sex roles and adaptive functioning of elders. Secondary objectives of the study included: exploration of antecedents and current experiences related to particular sex roles of adults; definition of the concepts of 'masculine' and 'feminine' as expressed in an older population; examination of the utility of standard measures, specifically the BSRI [1974], the Langner [1962] scale, the Philadelphia Geriatric Morale Scale [Lawton, 1975], and the Ammons Quick Test (QT) of Intelligence [Ammons and Ammons, 1979] as valid for older adult populations; comparison of older adults' perceived sex roles with the roles they believe are expected of them as men or women at this age; relation of sex roles and role complexity to decision-making styles; examination of the demographic factors associated with role choice, and application of information obtained to practical problems such as the clinical treatment of elders.

Research Questions and Hypotheses

Research Question 1:
Is the Older Adult Population at all Androgynous?
Age cross-sections of the population have been found to differ in the percentage of respondents who can be scored as high masculine/high feminine (or androgynous), high masculine, high feminine, or low masculine/low feminine (or undifferentiated). *Manning's* [1977] largely high-school population was mainly undifferentiated or androgynous, while *Bem's* [1975] college population was mainly sex-typed or androgynous. Rorschach data [*Ames* et al., 1954] suggest that normal older adults tend to score androgynously.

Hypothesis 1. Any cohort of older adults is predominantly androgynous in its sex-role orientation.

Alternative to Hypothesis 1. Factors derived from the BSRI differ in the current cohort of older adults on the basis of age and sex. While few factor analytic studies of the BSRI have been performed, it has been suggested by the literature that responses to the BSRI vary with both age and experience.

Research Question 2:
Does the Older Adult Who Incorporates a Multidimensional, Androgynous Sex Role Demonstrate a Different Pattern of Health and Symptomatology than One Who Incorporates a Simple, Polarized, or Undifferentiated Sex Role?
For example, women in general make disproportionate use of health services both of the physical health type and the mental health type. It has been noted that women become socialized into a dependent role, and that visits to a physician or mental-health clinician for help may be an expression of this role. If the sex-typed feminine role includes dependency, respondents scoring high feminine/low masculine should be more likely to seek help from a health service provider than those scoring high masculine, androgynous, or undifferentiated.

Hypothesis 2. Respondents who are sex-typed feminine make more visits to health service providers than do respondents sex-typed masculine or androgynous.

Alternative to Hypothesis 2. Increased health service provider visits lead to a dependent role, rather than flow from it. Since a direct investigation of this reverse hypothesis would require a follow-up study, a direct investigation is impractical at this time. A logical possibility is that health *mediates* the relationship between roles and visits.

Research Question 3:
How Do Respondents' Self-Reported Roles Compare with the Roles They Believe Others Expect of Them?

Several authors discuss the perceptions of older adults regarding age-related behavioral norms. They conclude that such norms exist, but may be expressed differently by different age groups. An individual may report behavior that is perceived as deviant from the consensual norm; in turn, perceived deviance from the norm can impact in interpersonal relations and on morale. Consequently, respondents were requested to respond to the BSRI to describe the sex-role attributes ascribed to them by people in general.

Hypothesis 3.1. Respondents project a consensus on the expected role attributes for older men and older women like themselves.

Hypothesis 3.2. Individuals whose *real self* role description varies significantly from the expected role description respond differently to several measures such as morale and symptomatology measures.

Research Question 4:
Do Sex-Typed, Androgynous, and Undifferentiated Respondents Differ in Their Descriptions of Current Situations, Past Significant Life Events, and Their Resolutions of Complex Situations?

Many studies indicate that life experiences partly determine the sex-role behaviors of a mature adult. Social-learning theory suggests that current sex roles expressed by older adults are learned from such experiences. The older adult who has combined roles in order to adapt to life crises is able to adapt in that manner during old age crises as well. If adult development stems from synthesizing the demands of developmental dimensional conflicts, as *Riegel* [1973] suggests, those persons who evolve complex solutions to life stresses will probably be the ones who have evolved either multifaceted, adaptive sex roles in response to conflicting societal/individual demands or polarized roles in response to the need for agentic or communal strategies.

Hypothesis 4. Members of sex-typed groups report different milestone events, differing recent life events, and differing styles of dealing with decisions.

Research Question 5:
Do Sex-Typed, Androgynous, and Undifferentiated Respondents Differ in Their Descriptions of the Complexity of Decision?
Multidimensional, flexible thinking is believed to be a general characteristic. Respondents who can coordinate several role aspects into a coherent, multidimensional role are expected to coordinate many aspects of a complex decision-making situation.

Hypothesis 5. Androgynous respondents report more complex multidimensional decisions than do either sex-typed or undifferentiated respondents.

Research Question 6:
Does the Androgynous Older Adult Age more Successfully (defined in chapter 7) *than Other Older Adults?*

Hypothesis 6. Androgynous older adults age more successfully than either the sex-typed or undifferentiated. Literature on personality and aging suggests that androgyny is associated with successful aging.

The study was intended to be more exploratory than definitive. If roles were not complex, neither learning nor a shift had occurred *or* the test was invalid for this age group. If life circumstances did not correlate with specific group membership, roles were not learned. If roles were complex *and* specific circumstances differed, either a dynamic [*Gutmann,* 1975] or a learning theory could be correct and could be tested further with this objective test. However, if roles were complex for only a portion of respondents and if roles were congruent with life circumstances, it is possible to argue that a dynamic explanation is not sufficient by itself. It will not be possible to disconfirm entirely a dynamic explanation for complex roles from these data unless all males score high masculine and all females score high feminine. Only longitudinal studies can adequately answer a question of role shift or lifetime learning.

7. Getting the Facts

Sample

The primary sample of respondents was made up of volunteers from selected Senior Centers of Maryland in suburban Baltimore and suburban Washington, DC. Centers were selected with the assistance of the Maryland State Department of Aging so that various economic, activity, racial, and religious groups would be represented. All 364 respondents lived in a community setting. In return for their time, a contribution of $5 was made to their center on the volunteer's behalf.

The sample utilized for the study cannot be considered nationally representative of the over-65 population. Respondents were participants at senior centers in the Baltimore, Maryland and Washington, DC Standard Metropolitan Statistical Areas (SMSA). Although centers from all ethnic and economic tracts within the two SMSA were contacted to participate in the study, only those centers where the Center Director volunteered were approached for respondent selection. Within these centers, volunteers were recruited as the respondents for the study. This self-selection process precludes generalizations of the findings to the national population.

The sample differed from the population of older Americans on several dimensions, but was similar on others. These are discussed in detail (population information is for 1975).

Sex. The majority of older persons in the USA are women, a pattern that was true for the sample. But while women comprise 59% of the over-65 population nationally, they accounted for 71% of the respondents in the study.

Marital Status. For elders in the USA, marital status differs dramatically by sex, largely as a result of differing mortality rates for men and women. While only 38% of women over 65 are married, almost 77%

of men still have a spouse. Conversely, more than half of older women are widowed and not remarried in comparison to only 14% of older men. Rates for remaining single, separation, and divorce are similar for women and men; remaining single, 5.8 and 4.7%, respectively; separation, 1.5 and 1.9%, respectively. The sample closely approximated the national norm.

Education. Nationally, older women tend to complete a higher level of education than men. 48% of women over 65 did not attend high school, 15% attended but did not graduate, and 22% obtained a high school diploma. The men exhibit a slightly lower educational achievement. 53% of men over 65 did not attend high school, 14% attended but did not graduate, and 17% earned a high school diploma. For those older adults who attended college, however, the trend reversed. Of the 16% of men who entered college, 9% graduated. Of the 14% of women who matriculated, only 6% completed 4 years. Respondents did not differ dramatically from the national norm. For men and women combined, 37% did not attend high school, 18% attended but did not graduate, 23% graduated from college, and 2.5% attended graduate school.

Ethnic and Racial Composition. Nationally, 87% of people over 65 are white, 7% are black, and 6% are Hispanic. Asian-Americans comprise less than 1% of the aging population. The sample was not representative in this regard. 95% of the respondents were white and 5% were black. Hispanics were not represented at all.

Income. Median income for older Americans is $7,300 although sex and race strongly influence this variable. White male heads of family have a median income of $7,400; white female heads of family have a median income of $ 8,500; black male heads of family have a median income of $5,000; and black female heads of family have a median income of $4,600. For elders in a nonfamily situation, median income level declines dramatically: for white males, it is $3,700; white females, $3,000; black males, $2,400; and black females, $2,000. Poverty levels for a 2-person aging family and individuals are $3,200 and $2,800, respectively. 15% of the elderly were living below the poverty level in 1975. The sample was not nationally representative in terms of income level. Median income for the sample was $6,000, slightly less than that of the population in general.

Age. Respondents ranged in age from 52 to 90. Mean age for males and females combined was 70.6 years. 45% of the respondents were 60–69 years; 46% were 70–79 years; and 33% were 80 years or older.

Living Arrangements. Living arrangements can be described in terms of four major categories: living with a spouse, living with other relatives, living alone, and living in an institution. The living arrangements of the general population of elders differ with regard to sex: 74% of males live with a spouse while only 36% of females reside with a marital partner; approximately 7% of males and 23% of females live with other relatives; 14% of males and 36% of females live alone; and slightly more than 4% of males and nearly 6% of females are in institutional settings.

Paid Employment. Nationally, older men display greater labor force participation than older women. 22% of men and 8% of women aged 65 or older are actively engaged in paid employment. The majority of respondents in our sample (90%) were not gainfully employed, although there was a high level (55%) of volunteer work performed.

Measures

The present study employed a wide range of measures. Included in the interview format were items designed to assess the individual's self-description of his or her own sex-role characteristics (BSRI), his or her conception of socially expected sex-role characteristics (BSRI with modified instructions), intelligence (Ammons QT), self-reported life events (open-ended life line), stressful life events (Social Readjustment Rating Scale), decision-making (tape ratings using Riegel's dialectical analysis), life satisfaction [*Lawton,* 1975], health status and the use of medication, mental health symptomatology [*Langner,* 1962], interpersonal relationships, demographic background, and an interviewer rating of the respondent's functioning and relationship to the interviewer. Each of these measurement devices will be discussed in turn, including their background and rationale for inclusion.

The Bem Sex-Role Inventory

The BSRI is a standardized, validated short inventory developed by *Bem* [1974] with the support of the National Institute of Mental Health. The language and length of the items, as well as its mode of development, make it suitable for assessing sex-role complexity.

The BSRI was administered twice, once with instructions to score the items 'as you really are now', and once with instructions to score the items 'as others expect you to be'. The BSRI contains a number of features that distinguish it from other commonly used masculinity-femininity scales. First, it includes both a masculinity and a femininity scale, each of which contains 20 personality characteristics. Second, because the BSRI was founded on a conception of the sex-typed person as someone who has internalized society's sex-typed standards of desirable behavior for men and women, these personality characteristics were selected as masculine or feminine on the basis of sex-typed social desirability and not on the basis of differential endorsement by males and females as most other inventories have done.

The BSRI asks a person to indicate on a 7-point scale how well each of the 60 masculine, feminine, and neutral personality characteristics describes himself or herself. The scale ranges from 1 ('never or almost never true') to 7 ('always or almost always true') and is labeled at each point. On the basis of his or her responses, each person receives three major scores: a masculinity score, a femininity score, and an androgyny score. In addition, a social desirability score can also be computed.

The masculinity and femininity scores indicate the extent to which a person endorses masculine and feminine personality characteristics as self-descriptive. Masculinity equals the mean self-rating for all endorsed masculine items, and femininity equals the mean self-rating for all endorsed feminine items. Both can range from 1 to 7. These two scores are logically independent; i.e. the structure of the test does not constrain them in any way, and they are free to vary independently.

The androgyny score is conceptualized as a reflection of the relative amounts of masculinity and femininity that the person included in his or her self-description and, as such, is thought to best characterize the nature of the person's total sex role. Currently, median splits are calculated on the masculine and feminine items and corresponding cut-offs are established for the sex-typed, androgynous, and indeterminate categories. The previous t-ratio method has been abandoned due to its inability to distinguish indeterminate types. This original method employed by *Bem* [1974] defined the androgyny score as the individual's t-ratio for the difference between masculine and feminine self-endorsement; i.e. the androgyny score was the difference between an individual's masculinity and femininity normalized with respect to the standard deviations of his or her masculinity and femininity scores. The t-ratio was employed, rather than a simple difference score, to assess whether a person's endorsement of masculine attributes differed significantly from his or her endorsement of feminine attributes and, if it did, to classify the person as significantly sex-typed in a particular direction. Also, different populations were able to be compared in terms of the percentage of significantly sex-typed individuals present within each. *Bem* [1974] employed this method in her original scale construction and validation described shortly.

Spence, et al. [1975] and *Strahan* [1975] pointed out measurement problems inherent in the t-ratio classification system. *Bem* [1975, 1979] and *Bem* et al. [1976] have accepted the new scoring method and have found it further strengthens their conceptualization. The new system allows for a 4-fold classification of individuals on the basis of masculine and feminine scores, but further provides, via median splits, a fourth category of individuals labeled undifferentiated or indeterminate (below the median cut-off on masculine and feminine scores), androgynous (above the cut-off on both), masculine (high on masculine, low on feminine), or feminine (high on feminine, low on masculine).

During the winter and spring of 1973, the BSRI was administered to 444 male and 279 female students in introductory psychology classes at Stanford University. It was also administered to an additional 117 male and 77 female paid volunteers at Foothill Junior College, Los Altos, California. The data that these students provided represent the normative data for the BSRI and, unless explicitly stated, they serve as the basis of all of the analyses that are discussed in this section.

In order to estimate the internal consistency of the BSRI, coefficient alpha was computed separately for the masculinity, femininity, and social desirability scores of the respondents in each of the two normative samples. The results showed all three scores to be highly reliable, both in the Stanford sample (masculinity = 0.86; femininity = 0.80; social desirability = 0.75) and in the Foothill sample (masculinity = 0.86; femininity = 0.82; social desirability = 0.70). Because the reliability of the androgyny t-ratio could not be calculated directly, coefficient alpha was computed for the highly correlated androgyny difference score, femininity-masculinity, using the formula for linear combinations. The reliability of the androgyny difference score was 0.85 for the Stanford sample and 0.86 for the Foothill sample.

The BSRI was administered for a second time to 28 males and 28 females from the Stanford normative sample. The second administration took place approximately 4 weeks after the first. During this second administration, respondents were told that the researchers were interested in how their responses might vary over time, and they were explicitly instructed not to try to remember how they had responded previously. Product-moment correlations were computed between the first and second administrations for the masculinity, femininity, androgyny, and social desirability scores. All four scores proved to be highly reliable over the 4-week interval (masculinity $r = 0.90$; femininity $r = 0.90$; androgyny $r = 0.93$; and social desirability $r = 0.89$).

The BSRI was selected for the present study for several reasons. A ratio scale, it locates people on a continuum from masculine to feminine. It is quick and easy to administer, as our pilot test results also indicate. It was developed using adults as respondents. The Institute for Sex Roles Study Conference (Ann Arbor, Michigan, June 1978) examined the concept of androgyny and the majority of participants reaffirmed their strong opinion that the BSRI was a very good, and possibly the best, measure of androgyny to date. The BSRI was pilot-tested with an elderly sample to verify that the questions are understandable to the population to be sampled in this study. *Gillett* et al. [1977] had earlier suggested that elders from 60 to 94 years of age had no difficulty in responding to the BSRI. Factor analyses of the BSRI [*Evanoski and Maher,* 1979; *Richardson* et al., 1979] have emphasized the conceptual clarity of employing factor-based scores labeled dominant/assertiveness, independence, and caring. Thus, the present study employed factor-analytic techniques to assess underlying factor structures. Scores on the BSRI have been related to diverse applications [*Beere,* 1979] such as family, cross-sex behavior, occupation, attitudes, conformity, mental health, anxiety, and cognitive complexity.

Beere [1979] reviewed 29 measures specifically addressed to adult sex roles. Of these, 3 were designed with androgyny implicit in their measurement: the BSRI, the Personal Attributes Questionnaire (PAQ) [*Spence* et al., 1974], and the PRF ANDRO scale [*Berzins,* et al., 1977, 1978]. The PRF ANDRO (1978) was compiled from items on *Jackson's* [1967] Personality Research Form (PRF). The instrument consists of 57 statements from the 400-

item PRF. Thus, researchers could ostensibly return to a previously gathered data base for reanalysis, or administer the ANDRO as part of a larger personality assessment picture, i.e. the PRF. Correlations with the BSRI ranged between 0.50 and 0.60.

The PAQ and BSRI correlations were 0.57 and 0.59 for males and females respectively on the female scale (F) and 0.75 and 0.73 for the male items (M) [*Spence and Helmreich,* 1978]. The PAQ provides subjects with a bipolar response format instead of a unipolar description. Since it is not clear whether the true bipolarity of traits such as independence-dependence was actually established empirically, this 'improvement' may be questionable. A second difference between the PAQ and BSRI involves item selection during the scale construction stage. Whereas *Bem* asked judges to choose traits more desirable for men and, separately, those adjectives more desirable for women, the PAQ items were judged by having raters specify the point on the same continuum of bipolar opposites along which the ideal member of each sex fell. Items that were judged desirable for *both* sexes, i.e. were on the same side of the midpoint of the scale, were chosen for consideration, and within this constraint those items that were statistically significant differentiators between the ideal man versus woman were retained for the respective scales. The M-F scale, unique to the PAQ, consisted of those remaining items that differentiated 'ideal man' from 'ideal woman' but were at opposite poles. *Spence and Helmreich* [1978] report that the M-F items in the BSRI M and F scales may confound studies on self-esteem. They retained the M-F scale separately to do justice to their conceptualization of M and F as attributes that are socially desirable in both sexes, but are more characteristic of one sex than the other. Unfortunately, to utilize the additional M-F scale, an 8-way classification must be derived from the 4-fold paradigm described earlier. While consideration of this issue seems warranted, the present researchers felt that *Bem's* conceptualization was simpler and tapped the variable of study sufficiently. Possible attenuation in BSRI construct validational studies does not impress the present researchers as being sufficient to warrant change at this point. Therefore, we chose to employ the BSRI because of the multitude of research available regarding its construct validity and reliability, including studies with older adults, and its simplicity of design and analysis. The PAQ and PRF ANDRO seem to be equally well-designed but are still relatively new in terms of the quantity of research employing them. In addition, *Bem* [1979] noted that her focus has been upon within-sex individual differences rather than between-sex differences in both item selection and validity studies, unlike the sex difference in the PAQ. As such, the BSRI does not presuppose sex differences on an a priori basis.

Ammons Quick Test of Intelligence

The question of finding good but brief instruments which can minimize fatigue in the elderly has been raised for intellectual testing. The brief test most used with the elderly is the Ammons QT [*Ammons and Ammons,* 1962, 1979; *Gendreau* et al., 1973; *Levine,* 1971]. The QT consists of three equivalent forms, each consisting of a single plate containing four line drawings and a list of 50 words graded from 'very easy' through 'twelfth grade plus' to 'hard'. The test is given by presenting a word to the respondent and asking him or her to select the picture which is most closely associated with the word. The QT has the advantage of correlating highly with the Wechsler Adult Intelligence Scale (WAIS), particularly with the WAIS Verbal IQ ($r = 0.876$ and 0.909, respectively). Normative data for a sample averaging 80.7 years of age indicate that scores do not vary with SES or years of institutionalization [*Schaie and Schaie,* 1977].

The scoring of the QT is objective and simple. The respondent is given credit for each item correctly answered. This scoring makes certain assumptions. First, it assumes that guessing has been effectively controlled by the tester. Second, it assumes that the respondent has been tested until he or she has failed six successive items, and until he has passed six successive items. The respondent is given credit for all items of difficulty below the six consecutive passes. A separate score is recorded for each of the three equivalent forms. Percentiles and Wechsler-type IQ norms are provided for adults, based on the assumption of a mean IQ of 100 and a standard deviation of 15 IQ points.

The short IQ measure was added to our study to determine the relationship among role flexibility, the mode of coping with life events, and intellectual ability. A short form was desirable so that the length of the entire assessment instrument would not be greater than other workable instruments we have used with elders in the past.

Open-Ended Life Line
Respondents were given the opportunity to respond to a completely open-ended life line. This simple measure was constructed to provide a useful indicator of the perception of milestone events by the cohort of elders under study. It was further hypothesized that a greater number of events might be linked to greater cognitive complexity or at least to a more eventful past. Historical milestones and developmental milestones have been suggested in many academic treatments of life events [see for example, *Davis and Brody,* 1979, p. 14], but the actual milestones as self-reported by older adults were lacking in the current literature.

Social Readjustment Rating Scale
The social readjustment rating scale (SRRS) was developed by *Holmes and Rahe* [1967] [see also *Holmes and Masuda,* 1964]. The scale was originally composed in an attempt to study the relationship between life changes and the occurrence of disease. Stress is the construct that is tapped, be it a positive event, such as a personal achievement, or a negative event, such as a divorce. *Sinnott and Guttmann* [1978 a, b] successfully employed a version of this scale in their research project on decision-making involving elders. In the present research, we employed the scale to ascertain stressful events that had occurred in the past year, in the past 5 years, and over a lifetime. Data analysis was performed only on events with the past year given the difficulty of retrospective data collection.

Tape Ratings
It is probable that experience in resolving issues surrounding major life events enhances an individual's ability to develop complex roles which facilitate adaptation in old age. Respondents were asked to select one major life event in which they may have experienced conflict or had to make a decision. In addition to administering the structured items just discussed, the interviewers probed for the nature of expressed conflicts and resolution strategies using a semi-clinical interview format [*Inhelder and Piaget,* 1958]. The responses to these inquiries (and only these responses) were taped and later rated by project staff who were blind to the other details of the respondent's profile. The theoretical basis for the choice of questions may be found in *Riegel* [1975, 1976] and *Sinnott and Guttmann* [1978 b].

Persons describing an event were analyzed in terms of four criteria: (1) the nature of the primary and secondary developmental dimensions of the event (biological, social, psychological, financial, environmental); (2) the presence or absence of conflict (thesis, antithesis); (3) whether the conflict was resolved, and (4) whether the resolution represented a synthesis of the two extremes of the conflict.

Responses were categorized by developmental dimensions according to the following five categories: (1) *biological* – health considerations (getting older, old and tired out, needed operation); (2) *psychological* – wants, needs (in terms of personality and continuity), emotional factors, stress, attitudes, intrapersonal events; (3) *social* – advice given by friends and relatives, institutional decisions or pressure, age-related expectations, housing arrangements and personal living environment, extrapersonal events; (4) *financial* – money matters, cost factors, ability to pay for services; (5) *environmental* – global events affecting the total population, such as war, changes in weather, deterioration of the environment. Responses were also categorized in terms of:

1. Conflict/No Conflict. Conflict was defined as opposition in the demands of two developmental dimensions. Three or four developmental dimensions may also be in conflict.

2. Resolution/No Resolution. Resolution was defined as solving the problem, making a decision, or arriving at an answer in some manner in regard to the life event in question. In unresolved conflict, on the other hand, the respondent is left fluctuating between the two (or more) oppositional dimensional demands.

3. Synthesis/Nonsynthesis. Synthesis was defined as the composition of oppositional parts into a more complex whole, such as the organization of species into genera. Synthesis is not merely the choice of one oppositional demand over the other(s).

We were interested in determining how many respondents experienced a major life event, considered several developmental dimensions in making decisions about that event, and described either a conflict, a resolution, or a synthesis, and which decisions related to androgyny as measured by the BSRI. Coping ability was hypothesized to be related to androgyny and to self-esteem, one measure of successful aging.

Subjects were also asked about their satisfaction or dissatisfaction regarding the outcome of the decision. Finally, they were given the opportunity to propose advice they might give someone else facing a similar decision today. These questions were designed to provide supplementary affective measures to the cognitive analysis.

Life Satisfaction
This group of items was composed of face-valid questions from the Philadelphia Geriatric Center Morale Scale [*Lawton,* 1975]. A factor analysis of the items indicated that they indeed measured high and low morale.

Health Status and Medication Use
Questions regarding health, in general terms, and the use of prescription drugs were derived from two prior Administration on Aging studies of decision-making and drug use [*Guttmann* et al., 1977].

Langner Scale of Mental Health Symptomatology

Langner's [1962] scale (labeled 'Survey of Feelings; B' in the instrument to minimize the possibility of defensiveness and social desirability in the respondent's answers) is designed to tap different operationalizable parameters of mental health. The available short measures of mental health symptomatology have been criticized on a number of grounds including: the utilization of items that are age-related; the social desirability of certain responses; and the inability of these instruments to differentiate precise symptomatology. As *Mechanic* [1975, p. 400] has noted, 'at present, there are no adequate reliable techniques for identifying psychiatric disorders in the general population'. *Gove and Gerkin* [1977] comment, however, that the utility of short-form measures of mental distress rests on their ability to provide comparative indications of general presence of symptoms among populations, rather than precise indications of illness states such as schizophrenia. With these cautions in mind, the research utilized the Langner scale. The Langner scale is the most widely used index of metal health symptomatology in community-dwelling populations. It has been shown to significantly discriminate between individuals independently described as psychiatrically sick or psychiatrically well [*Langner*, 1962].

Interpersonal Relationships

The 'Family, Friends, and Activities' section of the questionnaire was composed of relevant, face-valid items designed to measure the average number of interpersonal contacts made by respondents, either in person or by telephone.

Demographic Background

The 'Confidential Data Sheet' near the end of the protocol included logically relevant demographic data to assess such factors as SES, education, living arrangements, nationality, children, and work.

Interviewer Rating of Interviewed

The post-hoc rating by interviewers was included as an additional source of information regarding the respondent's degree of functioning and coherence during the interview. The eleven items came from the Philadelphia Medical School Clinical Gerontology Questionnaire [*Lawton*, 1975]. The scale was also used to eliminate respondents who were not capable of giving usable information.

Reliability and Validity

The reliability and validity data on the various standard measures used during the interview are discussed above in the sections which describe the instruments themselves. Coding-reliability estimates approached 100% intercoder agreement, and will therefore not be discussed further. Since interview items which were not standardized scales (for example, demographic items) had extremely high face-validity, the remainder of this section will concentrate on the interrater reliability on open-ended response items.

A coding system was devised for two sets of open-ended responses: significant milestone events in the respondent's life, and decision-making strategies. The significant milestone event analysis resulted in 22 possible milestones which could be present one or several times or absent for each case. Each milestone might be cited any number of times; for example, 'marriage' might be described as a milestone two times, a first marriage and a remarriage. 20 cases were recorded giving a possible 440 instances in which scores might disagree. Analyses revealed an 82% rate of agreement in scoring the milestone events.

The tape-recorded descriptions of respondents' decision-making in the most complex decision situation they had to face (as chosen by them) was also coded twice. The coding form was a modification of the original coding system [*Sinnott and Guttmann,* 1978 a, b]. Once again, 20 sets of responses were coded independently by two staff members. Interrater agreement on the primary dimension (20 possible points of agreement) was 90%. On the advice factor (20 possible points of agreement) agreement reached was 85%. Agreement on the secondary dimension (100 possible points of agreement) was 79%, and agreement of the 'result' factor (20 possible points of agreement) was 65%. Overall, agreement on the taped response codes (160 points of agreement) was 79%.

8. Life-Span Sex-Role Development Is Complex

Results were analyzed along the lines of the theoretical orientation of the study, as described in earlier chapters. Findings will be reported in seven subsections, as follows: evidence for a developmental stage of androgyny for elders; evidence for learned roles, due to elders' current life experiences; evidence for learned roles, due to elders' past significant experiences; evidence for the effect of social expectations on sex roles in older adults; relations between sex role and successful aging; characteristics of certain standard scales when used to test elders; and a summary of findings directly related to the hypotheses.

Role Complexity[2]

How do older adults characterize themselves on the standard BSRI? By using the median-split technique, it was found that 54% (197 persons, 71% female) were androgynous; 26% (97 persons, 88% female) were feminine; 9% (36 persons, 25% female) were masculine; and 9% (34 persons, 68% female) were undifferentiated. The androgynous and undifferentiated groups' ratios mirrored the sex ratio of the total sample, whereas masculine and feminine groups' ratios did not. Sex was controlled by weighting in further analyses using median-split groups.

By using the total-score technique, the extent to which the adults' M and F scores agree was determined. When total M and F scores were correlated by sex, Pearson product-moment correlations demonstrated significant M and F similarity for both men, $r(93) = 0.251$, $p = 0.0153$, and women, $r(222) = 0.246$, $p = 0.0002$, and explained 6.3% and 6.05% of the variance, respectively. Means and standard deviations appear in table I by sex. Individuals varied considerably in their endorsement of individual M and F items.

[2] Reprinted from *Sinnott* [1982] by permission of the *Journal of Gerontology*.

Table I. Comparison of *Bem* Sex-Role Inventory (BSRI) scores across age and sex

	F scores	M scores
Older adults		
Women		
M	5.35 (248[a])	4.39 (225[a])
Median	5.32	4.30
SD	0.48	0.80
Men		
M	5.01 (97[a])	4.95 (101[a])
Median	5.05	4.95
SD	0.51	0.79
Adult middle-class persons		
[*Hoffman and Fidell,* 1979]		
Women (n = 369)		
M	5.16	4.72
Median	5.20	4.74
SD	0.54	0.87
Men (n = 162)		
M	4.50	5.34
Median	4.52	5.38
SD	0.35	0.42
College students		
[*Bem,* 1974]		
Women (n = 356)		
M	5.03	4.57
Median		
SD	0.53	0.70
Men (n = 561)		
M	4.48	4.97
Median		
SD	0.57	0.68

[a] Number with complete scales.

By using the quartile (Q) split technique, the extent to which respondents' M and F scores agree was examined further. If a respondent scored in Q_1 on the F scale, a chance hypothesis suggested equal probabilities (1 ind 4) of scoring in Q_1, Q_2, Q_3, or Q_4 on the M scale. Of the 56 women in Q_1 on F, for example, only 14 (25%) would be expected to score in Q_1 on M by chance. In reality 45% of Q_{1F} women scored in Q_{1M} and 39% of Q_{1F} men scored in Q_{1M}. Those who scored low on F also tended to score low on M (37.5% of Q_{4F} women and 47.8% of Q_{4F} men). A χ^2 analysis was

Table II. Descriptive composition of principal component factors on the BSRI responses of elders[a]

Factor I: caring, mature	Factor II: macho
Sensitive to needs of others[b]	acts like a leader[b]
Self-reliant	(negative) feminine
Independent	masculine
Understanding	dominant
Affectionate	forceful
Compassionate	competitive
Warm	(negative) gentle
Self-sufficient	aggressive
Cheerful	
Strong personality	
Loyal	
Assertive	

[a] Unrotated; M and F items only; factor I – loads over ±0.45 only; factor II – loads over ±0.40 only.
[b] Ordered highest load first.

used to test whether, overall, agreement deviated from chance for men or women. In both cases significant results indicated that older adults reported equivalent M and F attributes; women, $\chi^2 (2) = 17.96$, $p < 0.001$; men, $\chi^2 (2) = 8.95$, $p < 0.02$. Effect size was moderate for women: $\lambda_{QF} = 0.25$; for men $\lambda_{QM} = 0.43$.

Comparison with Younger Groups

In table I is a summary comparison of three age groups' scores for descriptive purposes only, bearing in mind that both ages and generations are being compared at once. Longitudinal studies are critical in determining life-span changes. However, if there are no differences among groups, longitudinal studies with this standard test would be a waste of time.

College student scores in table I agree with other reports [e.g. *Bem*, 1975]. The average F scores are higher for older women and men than for their younger counterparts, except for the older men and adult women comparison. Older women's average M scores are lower than any other group's average M score, whereas older men's average M scores are lower than those for young men and equal to those of college men. The aver-

Table III. Composition of factors in the BSRI: responses of elders, after rotation, M and F items only

Factor I: communal	Factor II: agentic
Warm	acts like a leader
Gentle	competitive
Sympathetic	willing to take risks
Cheerful	athletic
Affectionate	aggressive
Loyal	ambitious
Independent	has leadership abilities
Tender	dominant
Sensitive to needs of others	forceful
Loves children	
Understanding	
Eager to soothe hurt feelings	

ages tend to mask the selective endorsement of individual M and F items by both men and women. This does not argue against a role shift for women; the older cohort most likely had a lower base M score in *their* youth than today's cohort of young women do. To summarize, there is evidence that older males and females describe complex male and female sex roles for themselves with men more balanced on M and F scores than women are.

Factor Analysis of Elders' Responses to BSRI

As *Whelton and Swindells* [1977] note, factor analyses of instruments proposing to measure separate male and female dimensions might result in a single bipolar factor, one masculine and one feminine factor, or several factors based on other traits. Factor analyses were performed to examine the response patterns of elders on this sex-role measure in order to make judgements regarding its validity for them. If the BSRI really measures something other than sex role for an elder group, their predominantly androgynous scores have little meaning.

Loadings from a principal components analysis, unrotated, produced 12 factors, only two accounting for 25.6% of the variance. The first factor might be named caring and mature, while the second is best described as macho (see table II). While these factors might raise some caution concerning what the BSRI is measuring in older adults, the varimax rotation of the factors, reported in table III, gives reason to believe that the BSRI is valid for this population. Although eight factors were extracted, only the first two, describing 53.3% of the variance, are reported here. Considering items with high loadings, the first factor appears communal in nature while the second appears agentic. Such findings are consistent with the conceptual nature of the BSRI and partially validate the instrument for elders.

Were the 20 so-called 'neutral' items on the BSRI really neutral for elders? In table IV is contained a summary of BSRI neutral items which correlate at least ±0.50 (relation describes 25% of the variance) with masculine or feminine subscale items. Selected neutral items are somewhat related to masculine or feminine items for every group. However, for the undifferentiated group there are 16 pairs with correlations of a magnitude greater than ±0.50, while the other groups have less. The conceptual space of the undifferentiated group concerning 'masculinity' and 'femininity' appears more complex in some ways than that of the androgynous or feminine, for which neutral items are mainly just that.

Do factor loadings on the BSRI vary by respondents' sex or age? The information presented in tables V and VI partially answers this question. For females, two principal component factors account for 51.6% of the variance and can be described as mature and caring (factor I) and 'aggressive' (factor II). After varimax rotation, the factors may best be described as 'communal' and 'agentic'. For males, the two main factors resulting from principal components analysis, after iterations, describe 43.9% of the variance and can best be described as 'compassionate leader' (factor I) and 'strong but gentle' (factor II). After varimax rotation, the factors may best be described as understanding and assertive but vulnerable. The pattern for females is more communal/agentic than that for males, but both tend to load in that conceptual direction.

Three factor analyses technically similar to those just described were performed for scores of respondents in their 60s, respondents in their 70s, and respondents 80 and over. For the 60-year-olds, two main factors accounted for 47% of the variance, and can be described as 'caring and independent' (factor I) and 'dominant and gentle' (factor II). After rotation, the two dimensions might be described as 'communal' and 'agentic'. For those in their 70s, unrotated main factors accounted for 49.3% of the variance and can be described as 'agentic/communal' (factor I) and 'leaderlike' (factor II). After rotation, the factors once again can be termed 'agentic' and 'communal'. For those in their 80s, three main factors described 46.1% of variance and can be described as 'leader-

Table IV. BSRI neutral item responses significantly related to masculine and feminine items at magnitudes of at least ±0.50, by group

	Neutral item	M/F item	Correlation
Androgynous group[a]	moody	cheerful	−0.53
Feminine group[b]	sincere	compassionate	0.70
	happy	cheerful	0.53
Masculine group[c]	conceited	self-sufficient	−0.51
	theatrical	willing to take a stand	0.50
	theatrical	aggressive	0.57
	theatrical	soft-spoken	−0.53
	helpful	understanding	0.54
	conscientious	self-sufficient	0.50
	conscientious	gullible	−0.54
	conscientious	self-reliant	0.54
	moody	gullible	0.60
	moody	cheerful	−0.65
Undifferentiated group[d]	friendly	warm	0.58
	friendly	tender	0.61
	unsystematic	athletic	−0.51
	tactful	ambitious	0.56
	conventional	soft spoken	−0.57
	reliable	childlike	0.54
	reliable	independent	0.52
	truthful	childlike	−0.80
	truthful	loyal	0.55
	truthful	sensitive to needs of others	0.71
	truthful	understanding	0.77
	truthful	athletic	−0.67
	likeable	gentle	0.53
	theatrical	athletic	0.53
	theatrical	gentle	−0.58
	theatrical	understanding	−0.53

[a] 18 other pairs correlated >0.32.
[b] 31 other pairs correlated >0.32.
[c] 55 other pairs correlated >0.32.
[d] 95 other pairs correlated >0.32.

like' (factor I), 'warm, affectionate' (factor II), and 'self-sufficient/sensitive' (factor III). After rotation, two factors ('communal' and 'agentic') once again emerge. Factor analyses, in general, confirm the dual trait nature of sex-role identity and offer evidence that the BSRI is valid for elders. Only small age-related and sex-related differences in factor pat-

Table V. BSRI items best describing varimax rotated factors, by sex of respondent

Females		Males	
Factor I	factor II	factor I	factor II
Gentle	acts as a leader	warm	competitive
Compassionate	competitive	sensitive to needs	athletic
Affectionate	strong personality	of others	gullible
Tender	forceful	compassionate	flatterable
Sympathetic	has leadership	cheerful	childlike
Eager to soothe	abilities	sympathetic	independent
hurt feelings	aggressive	understanding	defends beliefs
			assertive

Table VI. BSRI items best describing varimax rotated factors, by age of respondent

Factor I	Factor II
60–69 years	
Warm	dominant
Sensitive to needs of others	has leadership qualities
Compassionate	acts like a leader
Tender	competitive
Loves children	strong personality
70–79 years	
Gentle	acts like a leader
Sensitive to needs of others	competitive
Compassionate	aggressive
Loves children	has leadership ability
Sympathetic	makes decisions easily
Understanding	assertive
80+years	
No harsh language	willing to take a stand
Sensitive to needs of others	acts as a leader
Compassionate	willing to take risks
Childlike	masculine
Sympathetic	ambitious
Flatterable	has leadership ability
Feminine	forceful

terns are evident in the unrotated factors. The most noticeable differences include the element of vulnerability in the men's scores, and the degree of combination of agentic and communal characteristics in the age groups' scores.

The analyses reported so far suggest that most elders are androgynous, as measured by an instrument valid for elders, but that the factors or concepts underlying their responses may include more elements than those of 'agency' and 'communion'.

Correlates of Sex Roles

The second issue explored in this study is: 'Which personal and environmental characteristics, if any, are associated with sex roles?' Tables VII–IX summarize characteristics found to be significantly related to sex roles: median split (table VII), quartile split (table VIII), and total M and F score analyses (table IX). The footnotes indicate other variables that were analyzed and found to be nonsignificant. Tables VII–IX indicate whether men and women were analyzed together and whether scores were weighted to control for sex. Direction of causality cannot be assumed from these data with complete confidence since circular effects were possible. Many of the effect sizes were small.

Median-Split Technique

Masculine respondents tended to be married, feminine respondents tended to be unmarried, and androgynous-undifferentiated status was unrelated to marital status, χ^2 (3) = 15.26, p<0.001, estimated (est.) ω^2 = <0.01; effect for F, M, and undifferentiated groups alone = 0.39. Masculine and androgynous respondents had the highest incomes, and feminine and undifferentiated respondents had the lowest, χ^2 (3) = 15.26, p<0.001; est. ω^2 = <0.01; effect for F, M and undifferentiated groups alone = 0.16; for low income/high income groups alone, est. ω^2 = 0.25. Masculine and androgynous respondents volunteered to a lesser extent than feminine and undifferentiated respondents, F (3,509) = 6.12, p<0.01, but effect size was small (est. ω^2 = 0.01). The androgynous persons reported the best perceived health (compared with other older adults), χ^2 (3) = 11.84, p<0.01, est. ω^2 = <0.01. Masculine respondents visited doctors most frequently, F (3,509) = 5.02, p<0.01, est. ω^2 = 0.01. Mental health symptoms were most

Table VII. Summary of significant sex-role characteristics using the median-split technique[a]

	Androgynous	Feminine	Masculine	Undiffer-entiated
Sex	51% women	75% women	13% women	47% women
Marital status				
Married, %	49	37	75	47
Not now married, %	51	63	25	53
Income/month				
Less than $400, %	26	34	10	32
$401–$800, %	42	53	43	56
More than $800, %	31	9	47	12
Volunteering now	1.40	1.60	1.34	1.51
Health compared with older adults				
Better, %	77	58	69	59
Same or worse, %	24	42	32	41
Doctor visits/2 months	1.18	1.04	4.35	0.67
Mental health symptoms	7.59	9.94	8.42	7.54
Depression				
Always or sometimes, %	51	67	54	70
Never, %	49	33	46	30

[a] Entries are group means or percentages. Analyzed but not found to be significant: age; education; number of children or grandchildren; current working status; social interactions with family, relatives, friends; IQ; prescribed drugs used; psychotropics used; disability; milestone events; decision-making; nervousness. Weighted scores combined across sex. Some percentages do not sum to 100% due to rounding.

prevalent among feminine and masculine respondents, $F_{(3,509)} = 4.73$, $p < 0.01$, est. $\omega^2 = 0.01$, and the feminine and undifferentiated persons reported more frequent depression than the androgynous or masculine persons, $\chi^2 (3) = 9.34$, $p < 0.05$, est. $\omega^2 < 0.01$. Androgynous and undifferentiated respondents were equally likely to be male or female; feminine respondents were usually women; and masculine respondents were usually men, $F_{(3,509)} = 26.87$, $p < 0.001$, est. $\omega^2 = 0.05$.

Overall, the androgynous were notable for good perceived health, a comfortable economic situation, and not volunteering. The undifferentiated were notable for low incomes, few doctor visits, and depression. The feminine were notable for being unmarried, having low incomes, volunteering, depression, and having a greater number of mental health

Table VIII. Group means of significant sex-role characteristics using the 1st versus 4th quartile split technique[a]

	Androgynous	Feminine	Masculine	Undiffer-entiated
Years of school				
Women	10.48	9.80	11.31	9.29
Men	7.78	10.12	12.63	11.27
Ammons Quick Test				
Women	40.55	40.26	42.34	40.80
Men	38.89	38.44	43.22	40.64

[a] Analyzed but no significant effect for groups: mental and physical health; milestone events; decision-making; age; number of children. Small numbers precluded some analyses. Women and men analyzed separately.

Table IX. Summary of stepwise multiple regression prediction of total M or F scores for men and women[a]

Predictors for men and women	Relation to F scale total	Relation to M scale total
Men		
Years in school	negative	
Recent life event stress	positive	
Ammons Quick Test		positive
Doctor visits/2 months		positive
Depression		negative
R^2	0.179	0.143
Women		
Age	positive	
Number of children	positive	
Doctor visits/2 months		positive
Self-rated health		positive
Years in school		positive
R^2	0.046	0.079

[a] Analyzed but not found to be significant additions: income, disability, nervousness, drugs, mental symptoms. Scale precluded some analyses. Women and men analyzed separately.

symptoms. The masculine were notable for being married, high incomes, not volunteering, visiting doctors frequently, and having mental health symptoms other than depression. When considering major effects only, based on ω^2 and λ, the androgynous were characterized by higher incomes and sex balance; the undifferentiated were characterized by lower incomes and sex balance; the feminine were mainly poorer, unmarried women; and the masculine were mainly higher income married men. Results were not due to sex as an intervening variable as scores were weighted to control for sex. Discriminant function analysis [*Sinnott* et al., 1980] confirmed the importance of these potential predictors of group membership, which correctly predicted groups for 43% of the cases.

Quartile Splits

The advantage in using quartile splits (Q_1/Q_4) was better separation among groups; the disadvantage was a loss of respondents in the groups of interest, precluding some analyses. Sex by group comparisons resulting in significant differences are listed in table VIII. The masculine and androgynous women were found to be the best educated women; the masculine men were the best educated men, and the androgynous men were the least educated, F (3,167) = 3.68, p = 0.013, est. $\omega^2 = 0.02$. Ammons QT scores did not separate women, but masculine men had the highest QT among men, F (3,167) = 2.74, p = 0.044, est. $\omega^2 = 0.03$. Recent life-event stress was marginally significant: women reported low stress, and masculine women reported the lowest stress among women; men reported more stress, with feminine men reporting twice the recent stress of the masculine and undifferentiated and 50% more stress than the androgynous men, F (3,167) = 2.43, p = 0.066, est. $\omega^2 = 0.02$.

Overall, these Q-analyses pointed to new between-group differences and highlighted sex differences, but they did not always confirm differences found among median split groups. Fewer differences were found for women, other than masculine and androgynous women being well-educated and less stressful. Men differed more, with masculine men being high in education and comparatively low in stress, and androgynous or feminine men being less educated and more stressful.

Total M, Total F

An attempt was made to predict total M or F scores for men or women from their personal characteristics. Table IX summarizes the variables that made significant contributions to the prediction and states the direction of their relationship with either M or F. Men and women were analyzed separately. It was easier to predict scores for men than for women. The only new variable to appear significant was age, which had a positive relation with total F for women only. This might provide evidence of a sex by cohort underlying effect. Education was again an important variable: for men, the less school, the higher the F score; for women, the more school, the higher the M score. For both sexes health and doctor visits were associated with higher M scores. Effects for stress and IQ were unique to women: the more children, the higher the F score.

Overall, this third type of analysis appears to draw out sensitive sex and group differences without loss of respondents, although some variables could not be used due to incorrect scaling. It would appear from this type of analysis that the woman who is older, has more children, is in good health, and has had more education is the most likely to be androgynous, with her converse likely to be undifferentiated. The man who has little schooling, has high verbal IQ, much stress but little depression, and goes to the doctor often is most likely to be androgynous, with his converse most likely to be undifferentiated.

The three styles of analysis confirm the importance of some factors and present no contradictions. Some predictors appear cohort-related. Some of the differentiating characteristics (e.g. number of children, age, education) seem more likely to be partial causes of sex roles, whereas others could be both causes and results, operating in circular fashion.

Sex-Role Learning: Past Milestones

Mature individuals may be expressing sex roles learned from the impact of highly salient 'milestone' events in their past lives. How do milestones differ, if they do, for individuals in various groups? In table X are presented the significant milestone events reported by masculine and feminine respondents. Once again, it is supposed that significant events may have shaped the identities of these two groups so that they do not respond in the dominant androgynous manner. Masculine-typed respondents reported school, work, retirement, and historical events such as the Depression or World War II much more often than the feminine did. The feminine group reported deaths, marriage, and relations to spouse as milestones more often than the masculine did. Results here do

Table X. Mean number of milestone events by event type for masculine and feminine groups

Type of milestone event	Masculine group	Feminine group
Birth (respondent's)	0.06	0.05
School	1.08	0.55
Childhood	0.28	0.45
Marriage and relations to spouse	1.58	1.71
Children	1.33	2.05
Relatives	0.50	0.54
Work, paid or volunteer	2.44	1.03
Home	0.12	0.08
Present activities	0.33	0.29
Retirement	0.81	0.28
Travel	0.36	0.22
Deaths	0.69	1.29
Economic conditions	0.17	0.10
Friendships	0.03	0.07
Health	0.25	0.46
Historical/environmental	0.64	0.19
Lifelong avocations	0.14	0.04
Living arrangements	0.53	0.57
Religion	0.22	0.25
Special accomplishments	0.03	0.04
Philosophy	0.03	0.05
Mean events per respondent	11.47	10.33

support the idea that learning has taken place, but care should be taken in interpretation as sex was not controlled here and comparison has not been made as yet with the events of the androgynous group.

In general, some of the results reported in this section have supported the idea that past milestone events are related to present sex-type group. However, this trend is not a strong or clear one.

Age-Related Social Expectations for Sex Roles

Do mature adults perceive an overall age-related expectation about the sex-role attribute an older woman or man should display? Data in table XI can be used to address this question. Some general agreement exists (52.20% of respondents) that androgyny is expected of both male and female elders. The only other important expectation (overall, about 30% of respondents) is that elders should continue their polarized masculine or feminine role.

Table XI. Comparison of perceived sex role and social expectation for sex roles for female and male elders

| | Social expectation | | | |
	Androgynous	Feminine	Masculine	Undiffer-entiated
Females				
Actual sex roles				
Androgynous	97	25	6	11
Feminine	25	50	2	9
Masculine	5	0	3	1
Undifferentiated	9	10	2	2
	136	85	13	23
Percent	52.92	33.07	5.06	8.95
Males				
Actual sex roles				
Androgynous	39	2	11	5
Feminine	6	5	1	0
Masculine	8	2	15	2
Undifferentiated	1	1	3	6
	54	10	30	13
Percent	50.47	9.34	28.04	12.15

Data in table XI can also be used to compare the sex-role self-reports with social expectations. Approximately 60% of all respondents, both male and female, do not describe conflict between actual and expected roles. For the remaining 40% conflict mainly arises between sex-appropriate polarized roles and androgyny. For some the actual role is masculine or feminine while the perceived social expectation is androgyny; for an equal number the actual role is androgynous while the perceived expectation is of masculine or feminine traits.

Are there particular items in the BSRI which are the foci of conflict between actual roles and socially expected roles? The data in table XII may be used to answer this question. For androgynous respondents conflict (based on actual splits) almost never occurred on the masculine and feminine items (see superscript a in table XII) but was strong on two neutral items (superscript b). Other sex-type groups also had few

Table XII. Similarity of responses to BSRI under two sets of instructions: self-perception and social expectation

	Androgynous group	Feminine group	Masculine group	Undiffer-entiated group
Masculine items				
Willing to take a stand	0.1787	0.0265	0.4516	0.2324
Aggressive	0.3844	0.4577	0.4651	0.0751
Acts as a leader	0.3934	0.5451[a]	0.6185[a]	0.2076
Individualistic	0.1169	0.4384	0.5048[a]	0.0720
Competitive	0.3466	0.1736	0.3443	0.0277
Ambitious	0.2769	0.4031	0.2772	0.2096
Analytical	0.0834	0.0824	0.4722	0.1156
Has leadership abilities	0.3879	0.4266	0.3485	0.4854
Willing to take risks	0.3967	0.2574	0.2472	−0.1412
Makes decisions easily	0.1342	0.1378	0.4413	−0.0457
Self-sufficient	0.2187	0.1606	0.2152	0.3046
Dominant	0.3273	0.0782	0.6993[a]	−0.0903
Masculine	0.7386[a]	0.6213	0.6774[a]	0.7901[a]
Self-reliant	0.1493	0.2916	0.2305	0.3247
Defends own beliefs	0.1668	0.2278	0.3054	0.2377
Independent	0.2427	0.5507[a]	0.4536	0.4680
Athletic	0.6364[a]	0.5755[a]	0.5310[a]	0.7279[a]
Assertive	0.2023	0.3464	0.5918[a]	0.4460
Strong personality	0.3849	0.2649	0.2979	0.3652
Forceful	0.4388	0.2593	0.5556[a]	−0.0573
Neutral items				
Solemn	−0.5374[b]	−0.4228	−0.4493	0.5166[a]
Friendly	0.0890	0.1530	0.3355	0.0098
Inefficient	−0.2422	0.1707	0.1963	−0.2044
Adaptable	0.1721	0.1987	0.3451	0.2061
Unsystematic	−0.1511	−0.2381	−0.3761	0.5650[a]
Tactful	0.1010	0.0969	0.1529	0.1524
Conventional	−0.3449	−0.4016	−0.6821[b]	0.2962
Reliable	0.1316	0.2181	0.3491	0.2949
Jealous	−0.3194	−0.4466	−0.2573	0.1280
Truthful	0.1409	0.2523	0.4068	0.0873
Secretive	−0.4058	−0.4970[a]	−0.2541	0.5996[a]
Sincere	0.2157	0.2184	0.2765	−0.0155
Conceited	−0.3767	−0.1687	−0.3026	0.2541
Likeable	0.0284	0.1113	0.4614	0.2946
Helpful	0.0759	0.3017	0.2701	0.1465
Moody	−0.3025	−0.1972	−0.1748	0.6516[a]
Conscientious	0.1187	0.1775	0.4151	0.3653

Table XII. Continuation

	Androgynous group	Feminine group	Masculine group	Undiffer-entiated group
Theatrical	−0.7143[b]	−0.4723	−0.6884[a]	0.5225[a]
Happy	0.2253	0.4447	0.3041	0.5813[a]
Unpredictable	−0.4587	−0.5150[a]	−0.3654	0.3872
Feminine items				
Warm	0.1056	0.3336	0.4851	0.4386
Tender	0.3704	0.2176	0.0964	0.0938
Gullible	0.3017	0.2637	0.3175	0.2736
Childlike	0.3210	0.3053	0.2853	0.7414[a]
Does not use harsh language	0.3507	0.6106[a]	0.4502	0.2183
Loves children	0.0991	0.1607	0.3569	0.0665
Gentle	0.1450	0.1599	0.5503[a]	0.0767
Sympathetic	0.2343	0.2592	0.0202	0.0217
Sensitive to the needs of others	0.1766	0.3509	0.1786	0.1757
Understanding	0.0328	0.1086	0.1116	−0.1118
Compassionate	0.2189	0.1341	−0.0291	0.0516
Eager to soothe hurt feelings	0.2528	0.2817	0.0366	−0.0955
Soft-spoken	0.3491	0.3866	0.1168	0.6238[a]
Yielding	0.2295	0.2199	−0.1273	0.2555
Cheerful	0.0940	0.3548	0.2634	0.2723
Shy	0.4640	0.3859	−0.5086[b]	0.3056
Affectionate	0.3055	0.3097	−0.0571	0.1809
Flatterable	0.4216	0.4353	−0.1736	0.2053
Loyal	0.0325	0.3619	0.2016	0.2289
Feminine	0.7807[a]	0.7298[a]	0.0169	0.8635[a]

[a] Greatest similarity in response.
[b] Greatest dissimilarity in response.

Table XIII. Elements of most complicated life event[a]

	Androgynous %	Feminine %	Masculine %	Undiffer- entiated, %
Primary dimension				
Biological	15	9	1	4
Social	54	58	56	58
Psychological	8	11	14	15
Financial	9	7	10	5
Environmental	1	0	3	2
No response	13	15	16	16
Secondary dimension[b]				
Biological	33	44	29	44
Social	64	62	51	60
Psychological	67	58	42	55
Financial	34	32	43	49
Environmental	9	2	11	2
Outcome				
No resolution	24	23	20	25
Resolution without synthesis	33	46	36	20
Resolution with synthesis	39	28	41	50
Satisfactory				
No	22	19	16	21
Yes	67	63	78	72
Ambivalent	11	17	7	7

[a] Weighted to control for effect of sex.
[b] Not mutually exclusive categories.

strong predictors of conflict. Eventual discriminant function analyses may resolve the issue of which items best describe conflict between actual and expected roles [*Sinnott,* 1984 a–c].

Mental Health

Two additional questions came to mind. Is better mental health associated with congruence between sex and sex role? Is better mental health associated with instrumentality? To explore the first question, high M and low M respondents were separated and their symptomatology, nervousness, and depression scores were examined. Analysis of variance tests for M by sex effects related high M to positive mental health, F symptoms $(1,155) = 4.61$, $p = 0.033$, est. $\omega^2 = 0.02$; F nervous $(1,155) = 5.41$, $p = 0.021$, est. $\omega^2 = 0.03$; F depression $(1,155) = 8.19$, $p = 0.005$, est. $\omega^2 = 0.04$. Women had more symptoms, F $(1,155) = 9.50$, $p = 0.002$, est. $\omega^2 = 0.05$. To test whether congruence between sex and sex role had an effect, high F men and high M women were compared with high M men and high F women on the same three mental health variables. This time no significant effects were found. Claiming M attributes or balancing M and F were better predictors of positive mental health scores than having sex-role attributes congruent with one's sex, at least among these older adults. However, since avoiding disclosure is a traditional male attribute, too, high M persons might simply not report symptoms.

The next area of interest concerned the respondents' descriptions of their styles of coping with complicated events in their past, events which required that they make decisions. Do the androgynous resolve complicated coping situations more successfully than other groups do? In table XIII are displayed the dimensions of complicated life events encountered, the resolution of the event, and the respondents' satisfaction with the decision process and outcome. No differences among groups are apparent as far as dimensions of the event are concerned. In terms of outcome, the feminine group is unique in most often reporting resolution of the event but a resolution that does not meet all the demands of the event; other groups most often report resolution *with* such a synthesis. The feminine are the least satisfied with decision outcomes, while the masculine are most satisfied.

Support for Specific Hypotheses

The hypotheses of this study were largely supported. Each hypothesis will be briefly discussed in turn.

1. A cohort of older adults is primarily androgynous. This hypothesis was confirmed since the majority of the sample tested was androgynous in sex role. Factors obtained from analyses of BSRI responses, while qualitatively different in some respects from factors obtained for younger cohorts, did rotate to similar dimensions. No striking age or sex differences in factors were found.

2. Respondents typed feminine make more visits to health service providers than the androgynous or masculine respondents do. This hypothesis was not supported but its reverse was; i.e. masculine respondents made more visits while feminine made less, even with sex controlled. Perhaps there is a relation between agentic orientation and doctor visits. Health was not a mediator of the relationship described. A new alternative hypothesis, given these findings, might be that doctor visits lead to an agentic orientation, rather than flowing from it.

3. Respondents project a consensus on role attributes expected for older men and older women. This hypothesis was supported.

4. Individuals whose actual roles differ from their perceived socially expected roles respond differently to several measures, including morale and symptomatology. Only symptomatology was a significant factor related to sex-role strain or conflict.

5. Members of sex-type groups report different milestone events, differing recent life events, and differing resolution styles of complex decisions. Results were not clear-cut on this hypothesis. The reader is referred to results sections that are appropriate for summaries of a number of result patterns relating to this hypothesis.

6. Androgynous elders age more successfully than those of other groups. This hypothesis was supported, but not uniformly across every dimension of successful aging.

9. Adults and Society Adapt to Each Other's Systems over Time

The Bottom Line

First, how did older adults characterize themselves? In general, they outlined roles that usually were complex, with some respondents naming polar role-adjectives. Second, did life circumstances agree with sex-role descriptions? Life circumstances significantly differentiated the complex-role group from the M group and the F group, although some effects were small. Data therefore support the hypothesis that the objective test is valid (agreeing with *Gutmann's* [1975] cross-cultural findings), that sex-role shift may be a developmental tendency but not necessarily true for all older adults, and that learning is likely to play a part in sex roles in old age. The three methods each highlight different aspects of the interaction of sex roles, sex, and circumstances.

F scores were higher for males and females in this older cohort than for any other cohorts of males and females that have been studied. This is in accord with a role shift toward F for older men and does not preclude a shift toward M for older women. These older women born around 1900 probably claimed few if any M characteristics in their youth, in contrast to today's younger female cohort. Now, if they claim some M characteristics, they may have shifted toward M, even if they are the lowest cross-sectional cohort. Most older adults interviewed were dualistic in sex role as measured by the BSRI. For some, as *Garnets and Pleck* [1979] might predict, neither M nor F attributes were salient, although a balance was present. Those who were polarized masculine or feminine at the time of testing experienced a number of factors in their life that set them apart from the androgynous and undifferentiated. These factors (notably income and marital status but also number of children, volunteer work, IQ, education, and recent life stress) may constitute a learning experience that results in specific roles.

Besides the expectations that the BSRI is valid for older adults, that most older adults are androgynous, and that sex roles in old age are related to life circumstances, it was expected that, in general, a dual M/F androgynous role (whether a result of development or learning) would be associated with successful aging more strongly than polar sex roles would. This assumption, too, is supported: the androgynous group obtained more desirable scores on mental health items that are used as behavioral measures of successful aging. However, M was associated with desirable mental health scores more than F was [*Sinnott*, 1984 a–c]. A summary of the characteristics of androgynous, undifferentiated, feminine, and masculine older women and men, as determined by this study, appears in table XIV. The direction of causality between these characteristics and specific roles cannot be determined with certainty from these cross-sectional data, but it is unlikely that an old-age role shift from F to M made any older women's income high.

The androgynous and the undifferentiated respondents were very different from one another in terms of their table XIV characteristics. Androgynous women and men also differed. To speculate from a joint role-shift and learning position, the androgynous women seemed to be synthesizing roles to handle both instrumental and communal advantages (e.g. better education, more children), whereas androgynous men seemed to be synthesizing roles to deal with obstacles to instrumental advantages (e.g. high IQ but emotional demands of stresses, such as death, illness, and poor education) and to meet combined demands. The undifferentiated woman may be negating both male and female roles equally to deal with instrumental plus communal disadvantages she experiences (e.g. neither children nor education plus poor health), whereas the undifferentiated man may be negating both roles equally to cope with his somewhat unfavorable situation in spite of instrumental advantages (e.g. lower income and IQ in spite of better education) and fewer emotional demands (e.g. little life-event stress). There seemed to be few sex differences within the masculine and the feminine. Both sexes who had high scores on F and low scores on M seemed more stressed and disadvantaged; both sexes who had high M and low F scores had more of life's advantages. We speculate that older adults are ready for role synthesis and use it to deal with situational complexity, adjusting their investment in the dual male-female role (i.e. high investment equals androgynous; low investment equals undifferentiated) to reflect the anticipated success of masculine and feminine behaviors. They use polarized roles in less complex situations, although perhaps these roles are less adaptive in terms of mental health symptoms and depression. An

Table XIV. Summary of characteristics of androgynous, undifferentiated, feminine, and masculine older adults

Androgynous	Undifferentiated	Feminine	Masculine
Women			
Older[a]	younger[a]	older[a]	younger[a]
More children[a]	less children[a]	more children[a]	less children[a]
Better health[a]	poorer health[a]	poorer health[a]	better health[a]
Better educated[a]	less education[a]	less education[a]	better educated[a]
Less life-event stress[c]	fewer doctor visits[a]	fewer doctor visits[a]	more doctor visits[a]
Does not volunteer[b]	lower income[a, b]	unmarried now[a, b]	less life-event stress[c]
	more depressed[b]	lower income[a, b]	married now[a, b]
		more mental health symptoms[b]	higher income[a, b]
		more depressed[b]	more mental health symptoms[b]
Men			
Higher verbal IQ[a]	lower verbal IQ[a]	lower verbal IQ[a]	higher verbal IQ[a]
Less education[a]	better educated[a]	less education[a]	better educated[a]
More life-event stress[a]	less life-event stress[a]	much more life-event stress[a]	less life-event stress[a]
Less depressed[a]	more depressed[a]	more depressed[a]	less depression[a]
More doctor visits[a]	fewer doctor visits[a]	fewer doctor visits[a]	more doctor visits[a]
Does not volunteer[b]	lower income[a, b]	unmarried now[a, b]	married now[a, b]
Better health[b]		lower income[a, b]	higher income[a, b]
		more mental health symptoms[b]	does not volunteer[b]
			more mental health symptoms (other than depression)[b]

[a] Effect for this variable $\geq 5\%$ of variance for group membership; for stepwise multiple regression variable, added significantly to equation that accounted for $\geq 5\%$ of variance.
[b] From combined data of women and men, weighted to balance sex ratio. Might pertain more to one sex than to the other.
[c] Effect size less than 5%.

alternative explanation would be that these adults have set up long-term situations to match their chosen roles, but this seems less likely and would often preclude any age-related role shift. An over-the-life-span interaction between dynamic development and learning situations seems most probable and seems testable with an objective measure such as the BSRI.

Five Major Patterns of Sex Roles

Elder respondents displayed five major patterns of sex roles. It may prove useful to analyze the learning/successful aging patterns of respondents divided by these five patterns.

(1) Androgynous, unconflicted. These women and men scored androgynous, perceived that society expected them to be androgynous, and generally were not socialized to be stereotyped feminine or stereotyped masculine. Besides enjoying the generally positive aging of the androgynous group, they, as a group, would not be expected to suffer from conflict about their roles.

(2) Androgynous, conflicted. This group generally saw themselves as possessing a complex role, but experienced conflict about that role due to past milestone events, current life situations, or perceived social expectations which seemed to reinforce them for displaying only one aspect of their complex role. This group would enjoy the advantages of androgyny (if their behavior matched that role) while possibly suffering from the effects of conflict.

(3) Appropriate sex-type (men–masculine; women–feminine), no conflict. These individuals appear to be reinforced for a traditional sex role, perceived such a role to be appropriate for them, and identified with that role. While the experience of aging appeared less positive overall for these persons, they did not suffer from conflict.

(4) Masculine/feminine; sex-type inappropriate, conflicted. These individuals described themselves in traditional role terms, but terms that did not match their biological sex. Those experiencing conflict between expectations, reinforcements, and identity would be expected to show the greatest strain, although persons with an inappropriate sex-type are at risk of conflict under any circumstances.

(5) Undifferentiated. Apparently this was a group of complex individuals who may be beyond the androgynous stage (at some point of

sex-role transcendence), or may never have identified with any sex role. Some appeared to suffer conflict. More work needs to be done to separate the adaptive and maladaptive subgroups here.

Adaptiveness of Complex Roles: Individual and Species

Can it be argued that an androgynous, complex sex role is adaptive in some way for the individual elder or for today's society? Besides enjoying a wider variety of role responses with which to handle the sometimes conflicting biological, psychological, and social demands of old age, the androgynous person also has a means of counteracting the rigidification that often accompanies aging in this society. Choices may be fewer in old age, due to the larger number of choices already made, but some role options seem to open up wider than before. Roles such as sex roles might now be wide enough to allow specific, appropriate, targeted role responses which fit each situation. Looking at the sex roles of elders and comparing them with the sex roles of this same cohort when younger, one is struck by the fact that the period of 'rigid' sex-role behavior occurred in younger years.

Another adaptive feature for elders could be the control over others which complex roles can give them. They can articulate the rules and norms of several roles, but can be above conforming to them. If, instead, elders are completely caught up in stereotyped male or female roles, it is difficult for them to be the wise leaders who direct role development for all younger members of society. Role complexity both frees them and gives them power.

This point leads to the larger issue of the possible evolutionary significance of acceptance of complex roles in mature years. A population survives and changes both by putting limits on physical and behavioral variability, and by allowing for enough variability to occur for constructive change to take place. The individual varies within possible population parameters; the environment or society judges that variation to be worthwhile or not, adaptive or maladaptive. The acceptance of complex sex roles seems adaptive for individual elders; is it adaptive for the social system, too, or is it a variation that may be too extreme for society's own good? Is androgyny really a variation on basic masculine and feminine roles, or is it the *basic* sex-role tendency of which masculinity and feminity are variants?

The old in every society are the repositories of the basic, most important traditions of the culture. The young may use extreme behaviors, but the old with the traditional ways are always there to provide alternatives if the newer ways fail. Androgyny may be the basic, generic, integrated back-up sex role, kept intact by the mature generation, while the young produce the extreme variants of masculinity and femininity in response to pressures of courtship and reproduction. Now that more people survive reproduction to become old, the resurgence of this basic, generic role might become more evident. Traditional masculinity and femininity, sometimes considered signs of a basic identification that lasts through life, may really be like the momentary flourish of the peacock's resplendent tail – wonderful to see, fabulous for guaranteeing new generations, but something that gets in the way before and after courtship.

Developmental Theory: Which Theories Fit?

Results of the study speak directly to psychosocial theory, age-related expectation theory, dialectical, and Piagetian approaches. The two last will be discussed in a separate section, and the others below. *Erikson* [1963] suggested that older adults focus on the development of integrity, linking their life experiences into a meaningful whole. *Jung* [1933] theorized that dualistic aspects of personality would be balanced in old age. *Gutmann's* [1975] findings suggest balance between active and passive mastery for both women and men during this period. The finding that most older adults did combine dualistic feminine and masculine aspects in their self-perceptions and expected that elders do so supported the psychosocial contention.

Neugarten's [1968] age-related expectation or 'social-clock' approach also received support. This cohort of elders did perceive a general expectation concerning sex roles of older adults. Most of them conformed to the expectation. Further work needs to be done on the specific androgynous behaviors which are expected as age-appropriate, and on the actual behavior of elders in these specific situations. Do elders learn a different expectation and behavior if situated in a group with age-related expectations different from theirs? What effect might that conflict have in an experimental situation? Will this cohort be different from the next?

Riegel and Piaget. The developmental approach of *Riegel* [1976] proved useful in the conduct of this study. It opened the framework for analysis and conceptualization to include biological, social, psychological, and environmental aspects. *Riegel's* approach provided a framework for examining the interplay among several variables at different times in an individual's life, conflicts and variables which the individual synthesizes to adapt. Looking at behavior in old age as an outcome of (1) biological state and (2) resolution of past conflicts during past milestone events in (3) a particular historical setting helps resolve the occasional contradictions one finds between expected stage and actual behavior.

Riegel's approach unified aspects of diverse behaviors over time so that they could be examined as adaptive to the individual. This dialectical approach can be extended to examine the interplay between individual adaptation and species adaptation, and synthesis-resolving conflicts between the two. This study has not attempted to examine the adaptive value of androgyny for the species. But one might speculate that the postreproductive individual might still be adaptive to the species because he or she has the ability to integrate aspects of personality to serve as the balance for the group. Sex-role flexibility might then serve both species and individual through a complex synthesis of individual/group developmental dimensions. Biological, psychological, and social needs of individual and group would be jointly served in the current historical/environmental context.

Of course the next cohort of elders may need to strive for new adaptive individual and individual/group syntheses. The individual's biological situation may be different for an entire cohort, and learning from current situational demands or from perceived social age-related expectations might override an individual's developmental predispositions. A future cohort of elders might be the product of a post-World War III environment where increased population is needed. Childbearing and childrearing could continue far into later years, causing a biological demand and a learning experience favoring polarized sex roles. Under these new circumstances, an individual might be intellectually capable of androgyny but will display polarized roles in old age due to cohort learning experiences.

For another scenario, examine the case of young women in 1980 who do not perceive a biological demand for childbearing but do perceive an expectation for androgyny. If their experiences and cognitive complexity permit, they may assimilate the complex sex role earlier than the (currently) expected mature years, making an adaptive synthesis. If they are not psychologically ready to be androgynous in identity but learn the role due to circumstances, role strain and negative effects would be expected.

Piaget's theory [*Piaget and Kamii,* 1978] has recently been extended to explore cognitive development in everyday situations [*Sinnott,* 1975, 1983; *Sinnott and Guttmann,* 1978 a]. The ability to conceptually and logically combine masculinity and femininity into a complex, noncontradictory role (androgyny) and to apply that complex role to real situations may be one everyday measure of postformal operational thought in adults. Postformal operations, in this case, might be developed by adults who have gone beyond the formal operational stage, as described for the adolescent (where complex thought is hypothetical), and into the next stage where abstract thought is modified by being applied to reality [*Labouvie-Vief,* 1980; *Sinnott,* 1984 b]. In the case of this study, the reality involved social relations, an area of functioning where the cognitive operations of adults are most likely to grow [*Sinnott,* 1978, 1984 b]. Deeper analyses of the thinking processes of the androgynous respondents should prove fruitful in understanding one aspect of complex social-cognitive development and information processing of mature adults.

In chapter 2 we discussed a postformal concept of sex-role development. In it roles were not absolute but were created by individuals in an interaction. A belief about roles would be imposed on this system by the knowers, creating a somewhat subjective view of truth in this situation. This may be what many adults did as they responded to our interview questions, but this study was not designed to test this possibility. This study was not designed to examine role-taking as a problem-solving operation (see chapter 2), yet the flavor of the descriptions of persons in the four sex-type groups suggested that they may have used roles to solve life problems related to money, education, etc. More targeted studies are needed to examine sex-role taking as complex problem-solving.

Chapter 2 also contains a discussion of roles as connections between the person system and the social system. Although this study was not designed to explore the system approach to roles, it can be discussed in those terms. The study did point out the complexity of the information-processing system of the mature adults. This complexity was predicted by systems theory. Examining the systems models within the 'new' physics (chapter 2), we might begin to think of the person moving through developmental space and time in the company of other persons, like planets in a solar system. The gravitational fields of each planet/person influence the others and change their orbits, just as persons influence each other in families and societies. The perceived speed of development (or role change) and the direction traveled (or type of role developed) depend upon one's vantage point or view of the world. Is an elder masculine or feminine? In relation to which standards, those of society, himself or herself in past years, the ideal, the ideal in a context? If an elder is feminine, how can we talk about a 'cause' or 'effect' of that, without taking a whole 'solar' system of persons and the general-case laws of new physics relations into account? Systems operating on each other are known to move in interpenetrating realities to which linear models may not apply. We would be wise to take this into account in future studies.

In chapter 3 we made a case for the value of feminine response in maturity. Identification with a feminine, communal role appeared to be adaptive for males. We cannot say that the hypothesis of chapter 3, that femininity is adaptive in later life, has been adequately tested in this study, if for no other reason than we have not moved beyond the stereotypical definition of femininity, and have not specified a context in which adaptive behavior is being examined. This also awaits future work.

Many of the other issues addressed in chapters 4 and 5 and not discussed above were addressed but not resolved in the current study. Our measurement of masculinity and femininity was a measure of the stereotypic, sometimes negative traits meant to apply to general situations where the sexes are clearly different. This is one limited definition. We made links to behavior, but we cannot rest on the assumption that behavior in a given setting will be closely linked to any such limited definition. We created our own set of criteria for adaptivity, even though many others could have been used. Our criteria influenced the nature of the connection between roles and successful aging. Roles were assessed in two modes – real and expected. Older adults perceived expectations that they have complex roles, contrary to what others have found when they asked respondents to describe roles for generalized others. What did roles mean to our respondents? Again, future studies will be needed to answer this question, studies taking age and developmental stage into account. In this study change was assumed but not observed directly, and role *level* (not rate of change) was related to level of adaptation. Other models of viewing changes in roles over the life span are available and should be utilized.

Summary of the Study

We conducted a study of 364 community-dwelling mature adults, aged 60 and over, to determine (1) whether they generally describe themselves in androgynous sex-role terms or in nonandrogynous terms; (2) whether current life experiences, past milestone events, or perceived social expectations about roles might be related to described sex role; and (3) whether sex-role complexity is associated with successful aging. These research questions were embedded in a theoretical view of sex-role development in which the sex role adopted is adapted to the biological, psychological, social, and environmental contingencies experienced by the individual at a given life stage. Measures included the BSRI; standard assessment of verbal intelligence, mental health, physical health, morale, life event stress; and questions gathering information on milestone events, decision-making, and demographic data.

We determined that this cohort of older respondents was predominantly androgynous. The androgynous members experienced several recent life circumstances which differed from those of the masculine and feminine groups; some milestone events also seemed specific for masculine versus feminine groups. Elders most often displayed the sex role they believed society expected of them; those who displayed a role different from social expectation usually were appropriately sex-typed in the face of androgynous expectations or androgynous in the face of appropriately sex-typed expectations. On most measures the androgynous aged most successfully, although not all the comparisons were significant.

10. Methodological and Statistical Considerations in the Measurement of Sex Roles and Aging

The previous chapters of this volume have included some theoretically rich ideas regarding sex-role development in the adulthood and aged years, in addition to presenting the empirical findings of an ambitious study attempting to provide some initial support for such a challenging perspective. Perhaps the most salient notion that emerges from this material is that a confrontation with the complexity of human behavior is required to more adequately describe, explain, and understand sex-role development.

From a measurement point of view, the 'complexity challenge' requires the development and application of methodological and statistical tools that may enhance the probability of disentangling behavioral regularities from a multidimensional, dynamic context. The focus of the present chapter concerns one of the major psychometric issues in aging research, that of the comparability of measures. For example, how equivalent are the constructs of an instrument developed and normed on one age sample (e.g. college-aged) when applied to a sample differing in age (e.g. older adults). We use the sample case of the BSRI [*Bem*, 1974] in an application with an older adult sample to illustrate some of the issues involved. The presentation is not exhaustive of the multiple issues involved in the measurement of the complexly determined domain of sex roles and aging, but rather should be viewed as an exemplar of an approach to a specific measurement problem (that of measurement equivalence), as well as a demonstration of how the utilization of statistical models may facilitate inquiry into such issues.

After delineating some of the issues involved in the comparability of measurement, a data-analytic procedure, confirmatory factor analysis (CFA), is presented as a potentially useful method for assessing assumptions regarding comparability, and for hypothesis testing regarding developmental patterns. The CFA model is presented within the context of two other multivariate data-reduction techniques, principal components analysis, and common factor analysis. These three techniques are compared and contrasted with respect to underlying assumptions which have implications as to when they are appropriately applied.

A demonstration of confirmatory factor analysis is presented with data collected by *Sinnott* [1982] and analyzed secondarily by *Windle and Sinnott* [1985]. Suggestions are made for future applications of confirmatory analysis in sex roles and aging research.

Measurement Equivalence

Measurement equivalence is concerned with the likelihood that a given set of items, an experimental task, a behavioral observation, or any other method of measurement is tapping similar manifest or latent variables when applied to samples dissimilar on one or more dimensions (e.g. age) from the population upon which a given measure was constructed and possibly normed [*Labouvie,* 1980]. For example, if a measure is developed and evaluated on younger adults, it is not necessarily the case that the same instrument applied to older adults will measure identical psychological constructs. Some of the reasons why equivalence of measurement may not exist in developmental psychology include the possibility of maturational changes which may influence test performance, shifts in environmental contingencies which render constructs nonequivalent, and age by task interactions which confound the measurement equivalence of constructs.

Methodological issues surrounding measurement equivalence are not unique to developmental psychologists. Similar and in some ways more complex issues are confronted by cross-cultural behavioral scientists who have to contend with both different linguistic and cultural realities in the assessment of measurement equivalence [*Eckensberger,* 1973; *Frederiksen,* 1977]. A wide range of alternative methods of assessing the equivalence of measures have been proposed within this literature [*Frederiksen,* 1977], including the generation of equivalents, which are formally different but substantively the same as the identities of the original measure. This presumably provides a method of measuring identical psychological constructs with formally different stimuli.

In this chapter, we present an alternative, statistical method of determining measurement equivalence across multiple populations. This involves the comparison of patterns of covariation among items across samples on a self-report measure. The objective is to support the construct validity of the two-factor model for both male and female samples. Statistical significance tests are provided with this approach and indicate whether or not the internal structure of the self-report measure is equivalent for both samples.

Comparison of Three Multivariate Techniques

Before proceeding in some detail with the CFA procedure, it might be useful to briefly contrast this approach with more traditional multivariate data-reduction techniques such as principal components analysis (PC) and common factor analysis (CF). A commonality of the PC and CF approaches is to provide a more parsimonious description of the intercorrelations between a set of n variables with a set of F common factors or P components (with F and $P<n$). Both the PC and the CF approaches are referred to as exploratory procedures because the underlying structure of the data is not specified by the investigator. Rather, a number of decision rules (e.g. scree test) are used in the determination of the appropriate number of factors or components to extract, and rotational procedures are selected to provide a meaningful representation of the data. These two exploratory procedures are to be contrasted with the CFA approach, in which the investigator specifies (a) the number of factors in the data, (b) which variables are to load on which factors, (c) which factors are predicted to manifest salient or nonsalient (i.e. zero) relations with other factors, and (d) the nature of relationships among disturbance terms. Furthermore, the CFA approach offers a flexible and efficient procedure for testing hypotheses about the structure of data across multiple samples or multiple occasions of measurement [*Jöreskog*, 1971].

Although there are differences between the PC and CF approaches [e.g. see *Mulaik*, 1972], as well as differences between the similarities of these two approaches and the CFA approach, in some applications there is a convergence in regard to the selection of appropriate number of factors. In *Windle and Sinnott* [1985], maximum likelihood exploratory factor analyses were conducted on male and female samples. Maximum likelihood exploratory factor analysis is similar to the PC and CF models in that no underlying structure is specified by the investigator. However, the maximum likelihood estimation procedure is used in computations and statistical indices are provided regarding the fit of a given number of factors model. On the basis of statistical information provided by an alternative number of factor specifications, *Windle and Sinnott* [1985] selected an eight-factor model for males and a nine-factor model for females as providing an adequate structure of the BSRI for each sample.

Principal components analyses were subsequently conducted on the same data, and resulting eigenvalues and eigenvalue differences are reported in table XV. One of the most widely used criteria for determining the appropriate number of components (factors) in the principal components and common factor analytic literature is the root one criterion. This criterion suggests that the number of components (factors) should be equal to the number of eigenvalues greater than or equal to 1.0. However, this criterion tends to underestimate or overestimate the number of factors as a function of the number of variables, the number of factors, and the number of respondents [see *Gorsuch*, 1983, pp. 163–164 and references cited].

Cureton and D'Agostino [1983] have proposed an alternative criterion for determining the appropriate number of factors. They propose analyzing successive differences between eigenvalues until such differences are minimal, reflecting that additional factor extraction will yield trivial factors. The critical value proposed for determining the triviality of differences is approximately 0.15. Using this criterion to evaluate the eigenvalue differences for the two samples completing the BSRI, table XV provides additional, converging support for the eight-factor model for males and nine-factor model for females. Confirmatory factor analysis with a new sample would be required to validate eight- and nine-factor models, but this example demonstrates the potential convergence between maximum likelihood and more traditional approaches to factor analysis.

Confirmatory Analysis

The confirmatory factor-analytic model may be categorized as an example of a multitude of data-analytic strategies subsumed under the label of causal modeling, causal analysis, or structural equation modeling [*Bentler*, 1980; *James* et al., 1982]. Perhaps the major distinguishing feature of these data-analytic procedures, in contrast to others such as the analysis of variance or multiple regression analysis, is the model specification by the investigator of the causal linkages between variables

Table XV. Eigenvalues and differences for two samples, completing the BSRI

Factor	Males (n = 107)			Females (n = 257)		
	eigenvalue	difference[a]	percent of trace	eigenvalue	difference[a]	percent of trace
1	7.27		0.18	6.61		0.16
2	3.50	3.77	0.27	3.99	2.62	0.26
3	2.21	1.29	0.32	2.13	1.86	0.32
4	2.01	0.20	0.37	1.80	0.33	0.36
5	1.69	0.31	0.42	1.73	0.07	0.41
6	1.66	0.03	0.46	1.65	0.08	0.45
7	1.60	0.06	0.50	1.50	0.15	0.48
8	1.43	0.17	0.53	1.32	0.18	0.52
9	1.33	0.10	0.57	1.19	0.13	0.55
10	1.27	0.06	0.60	1.10	0.09	0.57
11	1.22	0.05	0.63	1.09	0.01	0.60
12	1.13	0.09	0.66	1.00	0.09	0.63
13	1.09	0.04	0.68	0.96	0.04	0.65
14	1.01	0.08	0.71	0.93	0.02	0.67
15	0.93	0.08	0.73	0.86	0.07	0.70

[a] Eigenvalues and eigenvalue differences were rounded separately. Consequently, reported differences will sometimes differ from the differences between rounded eigenvalues by ± 0.01.

within a system of variables. This specification includes both the identification of which variables are expected to relate to which variables, as well as which variables are not expected to relate to which variables. If variables within a system are not expected to manifest a relationship with one another (either directly or indirectly), a model may be specified so that these relationships are set, or fixed, to zero. The specification of the model also includes the freeing of parameters where relationships are expected to exist among variables. The testing of the model consists of obtaining estimates for the freed parameters of the specified model and evaluating the adequacy, plausibility, or fit of the model according to various statistical information (e.g. χ^2 statistic/d.f.). Statistical goodness of fit refers to the likelihood that the specified, or hypothesized, model adequately reproduces the observed data (more specifically, the observed variance/covariance matrix).

The application of causal modeling techniques has been much more prevalent in the econometrics and sociological literature [for historical review, see *Bentler,* 1980]. Recent advances in cost-efficient parameter estimation algorithms have facilitated the viability of using such techniques and have contributed to its utilization within these disciplines and its expansion to others, including psychology. One of the most widely used computer programs in structural equation modeling is LISREL-V [*Jöreskog and Sörbom,* 1981], or one of its predecessors (e.g. COFAMM). LISREL-V enables the researcher to specify a model regarding the predicted relationships among variables, provides efficient and consistent maximum likelihood estimates for the parameters to be estimated, and yields output regarding the statistical fit of the model as well as identifying where the specified models need to be adjusted (i.e. what parameter constraints need to be relaxed) to obtain a better fitting model. *Muthen's* [1984] LACCI program, which uses generalized least squares estimation, also holds considerable promise in future applications of structural equation modeling, due to the flexibility in simultaneously handling categorical and continuous variables.

In the present chapter we confine ourselves to LISREL-V and to confirmatory factor-analytic applications. Within the literature on LISREL [e.g. *Jöreskog and Sörbom,* 1979], these applications are concerned with the measurement model, or the internal structure of measures. The measurement model is distinguished from the structural equation model in that the latter is concerned with the causal relations between a system of latent and possibly manifest variables, including parameter estimates of regression coefficients between variables. Our example will focus on using LISREL-V to establish construct validity for two factors of the BSRI [*Bem,* 1974].

Research Applications

The data used in this illustration of the application of LISREL-V to sex roles and aging were collected by *Sinnott* and reported in the present volume. The sample was representative of the national older adult population in several ways, including comparable frequencies in categories of sex, marital status, and race, as well as similar mean levels and standard deviations for income and educational attainment. The data of 257 women and 107 men are used in this illustration. (For more details on sample characteristics and the methodology, see chapter 7.) The mean age of the total sample was 70.6 years (range 60–90).

Windle and Sinnott [1985] performed a secondary analysis on the data collected by *Sinnott* [1982], with a focus on the dimensional structure of the BSRI for older adults. Two of the major findings that emerged from the secondary analysis were that the two-factor orthogonal model of the BSRI did not adequately represent the structure of the covariance matrices for these samples, and that the underlying factorial structure of the BSRI differed for males and females. Subsequent exploratory factor analyses for these samples with a maximum likelihood exploratory factor-analytic program [*Jöreskog and Sorbom*, 1978] yielded an eight-factor model for males, and a nine-factor model for females.[3] There was substantial overlap among five factors for the two samples.

In the example provided, indicators (items) of two factors which displayed similar item-factor relations across male and female samples are abstracted from the total complement of items on the BSRI, and hypotheses are tested regarding factorial invariance across groups. We are, of course, capitalizing on the findings from the exploratory factor analyses, and relationships regarding factorial invariance need to be cross-validated on a different sample. However, this example is intended to be illustrative of a way one might proceed to test hypotheses regarding the underlying structure of a given data set, and how one might make simultaneous comparisons with multiple samples.

Ten items from the BSRI were selected for the specification of a two-factor model. Six of the items manifested high loadings in the exploratory factor-analyses by *Windle and Sinnott* [1985] for both males and females, and the factor was labeled masculine/competent. Similarly, the other four items loaded high for both samples on a factor labeled femininity. The LISREL model specification for the ten-item, two-factor model is presented in figure 3. The two columns in Λ_y represent the hypothesized structure of the factor loading pattern, with Λ_1–Λ_6 corresponding to items 1–6, and Λ_7–Λ_{10} corresponding to items 7–10. Parameter estimates are sought for each of the ten Λ_s. Note that zeroes are

---

[3] In defense of the BSRI, it should be noted that at the time of its development maximum likelihood factor-analytic programs were not widely distributed nor frequently used by nonstatisticians. There are still many unanswered questions concerning the utilization of these procedures in applications with large item inventories, and it is highly probable that a 'good statistical fit' would be difficult to obtain with many of our most widely used measures (e.g. WAIS, 16 PF).

$$\Lambda_y = \begin{bmatrix} \lambda_1 & 0 \\ \lambda_2 & 0 \\ \lambda_3 & 0 \\ \lambda_4 & 0 \\ \lambda_5 & 0 \\ \lambda_6 & 0 \\ 0 & \lambda_7 \\ 0 & \lambda_8 \\ 0 & \lambda_9 \\ 0 & \lambda_{10} \end{bmatrix}$$

$$\Psi = \begin{bmatrix} 1 & \\ \psi_1 & 1 \end{bmatrix}$$

$$\Theta_\varepsilon = \begin{bmatrix} \varepsilon_1 \\ 0 & \varepsilon_2 \\ 0 & 0 & \varepsilon_3 \\ 0 & 0 & 0 & \varepsilon_4 \\ 0 & 0 & 0 & 0 & \varepsilon_5 \\ 0 & 0 & 0 & 0 & 0 & \varepsilon_6 \\ 0 & 0 & 0 & 0 & 0 & 0 & \varepsilon_7 \\ 0 & 0 & 0 & 0 & 0 & 0 & 0 & \varepsilon_8 \\ 0 & 0 & 0 & 0 & 0 & 0 & 0 & 0 & \varepsilon_9 \\ 0 & 0 & 0 & 0 & 0 & 0 & 0 & 0 & 0 & \varepsilon_{10} \end{bmatrix}$$

Fig. 3. LISREL specification for two-factor model of BSRI traits

specified for all of the other elements in Λ_y, indicating that no relationships, or nonsignificant loadings, are predicted for each of these item-factor relations (e.g. item one is constrained to zero and not permitted to load on factor 2). The factor intercorrelation matrix (ψ) has two fixed values along its diagonal, and a freed parameter to be estimated which corresponds to the intercorrelation between factors one and two. The two diagonal elements of ψ are arbitrarily fixed to one to establish a common metric for the factors. Parameter estimates for the disturbance term for each of the items is specified in the diagonal matrix Θ_ε. Disturbance terms are assumed to be uncorrelated with one another, and therefore all off-diagonal elements in Θ_ε are fixed to zero.

The specified two-factor LISREL model was run separately for males and females. The χ^2 statistic for males was 38.83 with 34 degrees of freedom (p = 0.26), and for females was 49.60 with 34 degrees of freedom (p = 0.04). Given these findings, we cannot reject the plausibility of the two-factor model for either sample. The standardized factor-analytic solution for each sample is presented in table XVI and XVII.

In analyzing these two tables, observe the similarities in the magnitude and rank-ordering of the factor loadings across samples. Even though *Windle and Sinnott* [1985] reported significant differences between genders in testing the omnibus hypothesis regarding the equality of covariance matrices across genders, it is possible to test for partial invariance for component matrices (e.g. Λ), or for a subset of factors. That is, it is possible to have a partially homogeneous, partially heterogeneous latent structure across populations.

Jöreskog [1971] and *Alwin and Jackson* [1981] have proposed sequential hypothesis-testing procedures to assess factorial invariance in multiple group designs. Table XVIII summarizes this sequence of hypotheses testing for the ten-item, two-factor structure of the BSRI for the male and female samples.[4] Goodness of fit information for the single group models is reported in the upper portion of table XVIII. The simultaneous group models included specifications of varying degrees of invariance across samples, with all parameters, for both groups estimated simultaneously (in contrast to single group models in which parameters are estimated separately for each group). In making simultaneous group comparisons, it is necessary to use covariance matrices, rather than correlation matrices, since the standardization of the latter may distort significant differences in variances and covariances between samples.[5]

Model 1 provided a test of the omnibus hypothesis that the variance/covariance matrices for the two samples were equal. The associated probability level for this model indicates that this is not a plausible

---

[4] In order to more adequately test the hypothesis that the masculine/competent and femininity factors are invariant across samples, it would be necessary to specify such a model with all forty items of the BSRI masculinity and femininity subscales. This would be necessary because LISREL-V uses full information maximum likelihood estimation, meaning that all parameters in the model are estimated simultaneously. Therefore, the parameter estimates and fit statistics obtained for our subset of ten items may take on different values when estimated within the context of all 40 items.

[5] Covariance matrices, as well as correlational matrices for the ten items used in this sample, are available from the author upon request.

Table XVI. Standardized solution for two-factor model of BSRI traits for males (n = 107)

Items	Masculine/competent	Feminine
Defends own beliefs	0.47	0.00
Analytical	0.44	0.00
Makes decisions easily	0.56	0.00
Self-sufficient	0.24	0.00
Willing to take a stand	0.47	0.00
Acts as a leader	0.73	0.00
Yielding	0.00	0.33
Shy	0.00	0.83
Flatterable	0.00	0.33
Sympathetic	0.00	0.85
Factor intercorrelations	1.00	
	0.32	1.00

The specified model yielded the following statistical information: χ^2 statistic = 38.83, d.f. = 34, p > 0.25.

Table XVII. Standardized solution for two-factor model of BSRI traits for females (n = 257)

Items	Masculine/competent	Feminine
Defends own beliefs	0.63	0.00
Analytical	0.53	0.00
Makes decisions easily	0.61	0.00
Self-sufficient	0.51	0.00
Willing to take a stand	0.48	0.00
Acts as a leader	0.78	0.00
Yielding	0.00	0.33
Shy	0.00	0.81
Flatterable	0.00	0.48
Sympathetic	0.00	0.85
Factor intercorrelations	1.00	
	0.09	1.00

The specified model yielded the following statistical information: χ^2 statistic = 49.60, d.f. = 34, p > 0.04.

Table XVIII. Goodness of fit information for single- and simultaneous-group factor models

Model	χ^2 statistic	d.f.	Prob. level
Single-group models			
Males	38.83	34	0.26
Females	49.60	34	0.04
Sum	88.43	68	
Simultaneous-group models			
1 $\Sigma_M = \Sigma_F$	91.05	55	0.00
2 $\Lambda_M = \Lambda_F$	92.08	76	0.10
3 $\Lambda_M = \Lambda_F$; $\Psi_M = \Psi_F$	132.30	86	0.00
4 $\Lambda_M = \Lambda_F$; $\Theta_M = \Theta_F$	96.59	79	0.09
5 $\Lambda_M = \Lambda_F$; $\Theta_M = \Theta_F$; $\Psi_M = \Psi_F$	135.68	89	0.00

The symbols referred to in the simultaneous-group models correspond to the covariance (correlation) structure equation $\Sigma = \Lambda\Theta\Lambda^1 + \Psi^2$, where Σ = covariance matrix; Λ = factor regression matrix; Θ = covariance matrix for the latent factors; and Ψ^2 = diagonal matrix of disturbances.

hypothesis, and that the samples differ. To test for the invariance of just the factor loading pattern, *Alwin and Jackson* [1981] proposed testing the difference between the statistical information obtained for a simultaneous model specified to have factor loading equivalence across groups, with the statistical information obtained from the sum of the single group models. That is, the single group models provide an adequate fit and similar factor loading patterns for both samples. The specification in model 2 tests whether it is plausible that the factor loadings can be simultaneously estimated to be equal across samples. The probability level associated with model 2 suggests that the model fits the data, and the difference obtained by the Alwin-Jackson comparison is 3.65 with eight degrees of freedom (i.e. 92.08–88.43; 76–68), further supporting the plausibility of the invariance of the factor loading pattern across samples.

Given the invariance of the factor loading pattern, it is appropriate to proceed to test for invariance in additional parameter matrices. Model 3 tested the hypothesis of equal factor loadings and equal disturbance terms across samples. The associated probability level indicated that this was not a plausible hypothesis. Furthermore, *Alwin and Jackson* [1981] suggest that the statistical information of a model 3 specification be compared with that of a model 2 specification. The difference between these two models is 40.22 with 10 degrees of freedom (i.e. 132.30–92.08; 86–76), indicating the inadequacy of fit. The model 4 specification tested the hypothesis that the factor loading patterns and the factor intercorrelation matrices were equal across samples. This hypothesis could not be rejected since the difference between models was 4.51 with three degrees of freedom (i.e. 96.59–92.08; 79–76), and the associated probability level was 0.09. Model 5 provided a test for the invariance of all three parameter matrices across samples. Neither the associated probability level nor the difference between model 5 and model 4 supported the plausibility of the invariance hypothesis of model 5.

In summary, the sequential hypothesis testing procedure revealed a factorially invariant structure for the BSRI for male and female samples in the factor regression (loading) matrices and in the covariance matrices of the latent factors. Differences were found between samples in the diagonal matrix of disturbances. The hypothesis testing procedure used in this example may provide a method of assessing similarities and differences between genders, between groups of different ages, and between performances by the same individuals on multiple occasions of measurement.

Summary and Future Directions

The principal intent of this chapter was to identify a major psychometric issue in the study of development and aging, that of measurement equivalence, and to propose an analytical strategy to deal with it. Data on sex roles and aging were used to illustrate how one might proceed to test alternative hypotheses about the underlying factorial structure of a measure for multiple samples. LISREL-V was introduced and utilized in the assessment of varying degrees of factorial invariance across samples of older adult males and females. Factorial invariance was found for the factor loading patterns and the intercorrelation matrices for the two samples.

While the application of confirmatory factor analysis in the present article was limited to similarities and differences between genders of older adults, it has potential for assessing similarities and differences among age groups and to test theoretical expectations regarding developmental change phenomena. As mentioned briefly by *Windle and Sin-*

nott [1985], the confirmatory factor analytic model could be used to test structural developmental theories of sex-role changes in personality functioning concomitant with aging. Initial efforts would involve the collection of data from multiple age groups completing the BSRI and applying exploratory data analytic procedures to see if (a) factors appear to differentiate with aging (as indicated by a greater number of factors to account for the data among the aged), or (b) the pattern of factor inter-correlations changes, or (c) factors differentiate and factor intercorre-lations change. If one of these patterns was observed, it would be possible to collect data on new samples and specify models which test the hypothesized patterns of covariation. Sequential research designs could also be used to facilitate the interpretation of one's findings regarding development and change [*Schaie,* 1977].

Michael T. Windle

11. The Next Steps

The purpose of this book was to consolidate and briefly present recent empirical and theoretical work on sex-role development in mature adults. The major focus has been on roles in men and women over 60 years of age. An additional purpose has been to interpret recent work and to suggest ways in which ideas in other fields – sociobiology, systems theory, cognitive psychology, and the new physics, for example – can be used to give meaning to sex-role development. Admittedly, these purposes can be achieved only in a limited way in this short presentation. But this book has represented an attempt to stimulate thinking and to bridge disciplines as well as areas within psychology.

The subtitle of the book – *Theory and Research from a Systems Perspective* – reflects the author's overall concern that we study and talk about the developing person *in context.* However, most of the work on sex roles is not done in this systems frame of reference. Only a few thinkers focus on one system or another, but usually they do not say they are systems-oriented or they do not use the language of general systems theory. What would seem most useful to researchers is to remember that at all points in the life span the personal and the social systems intersect and influence each other, and that each also tries to maintain a continuity over time. Sex roles are one intersection. The dynamic tension represented by this multisystem process may be expressing itself in the reports of sex-role behavior which we have seen. Many theorists touch upon one or the other portions of the process, but do not acknowledge the whole. When we acknowledge the whole process we see how biology, knowledge, action, feeling, belief, perception, stereotype, standards, and time co-construct this part of the interpersonal world.

Roles Are Possibilities for Action

Emerging ideas suggest that in the future roles will be orchestrated consciously by the person, rather than being imposed by society, or being left to the mercy of unexamined forces. Each child may grow up aware that he or she has a spectrum of role possibilities within, a cast of characters and a library of dramas which can be played out. The child will see that at some times in life one character or one drama is more useful than the others and so can be invited into life. The child will be aware that using only one character or drama can be habit-forming, and that alternatives should be practiced so that they are ready for use as desired. This child will remember, even before old age, that these characters and dramas are only roles, not his or her entire self, and that each person has much greater potential than can ever be confined within a role framework. After all, we are an emerging species, or we are a dying species. That child will see that change is expected, and as good a representation of life as is continuity. The child will be aware that maleness and femaleness are only what we decide they are. If peers communicate expectations, those expectations can be consciously and calmly met, or not, as a matter of choice. This child of the future can then remind others that they too can be more, that they are potentially all the characters, that they can act in all the dramas. So the author predicts that roles will soon come to be seen as a reflection of personal problem-solving styles. This will create a more flexible social organism, in turn, after transitional upheaval and reaction to that upheaval are finished.

Recapitulation

In this book we have explored the evolution of sex-role theory, noting the factors that made it likely that we would be interested, today, in sex-role development in older adults. Conceptualizations of sex roles have been a function of philosophy, history, economics, and politics. Researchers study what seems important at the time. Roles have been conceptualized as developing (or unfolding), as learned via social encounters, or as enacted after cognitive assimilation of a role concept in childhood. The relatively recent life-span approach incorporates all of the above dimensions. Measures of masculine and feminine roles have reflected the transition from seeing roles as general concrete entities on a single continuum to thinking of them as multicaused, multifactor concepts of certain salience at some life-span point.

We explored some new life-span approaches which focused on the developing person in the developing social system: Piagetian postformal cognitive operations; dialectical theory, and systems theory. When we examine sex roles in the context of cognitive functioning or in the contexts of sociobiological approaches or of history, we notice that roles seem to be components of systems that operate in almost organic ways. Like the living systems of *Miller* [1978], these systems use roles to make contact between individuals and larger systems, and to spur change or meet crises for adaptation purposes. Examining sex roles in context raises questions about the narrow ways they are typically conceptualized and suggests new research approaches that are broader in scope.

We examined roles from an evolutionary perspective considering some species-related factors in older adults' role transformations. Successful adaptation to the environment becomes increasingly important with aging but the ability to adapt may depend upon already having certain traits, skills, and attributes, many of which are communal in nature. The valuing of communal traits by our culture must increase if people are to pass through old age successfully. Then we can all share *Bakan's* [1966] vision that the 'proper way of dying is from fatigue after a life of trying to mitigate agency with communion' (p. 236).

Recent literature leads to considerations for future research on sex roles in mature adults, or in adults of any age. In general, recent theoretical work has demonstrated the complexities of reaching a meaningful measurement of masculinity, femininity, androgyny, adjustment, or self-concept. Few investigators can hope to address all the issues raised, but more can be conscious of them in interpreting data. Together, all of the authors seemed to be urging use of a complex model for change and for any role-related behavior. The perceptions of the respondent – about the meaning of items, about social sanctions, about situational salience – stand out as factors to be attended to in future work as soon as means can be found to measure them. Researchers considered the nature of adaptivity in a social setting; social approval and disapproval of role-related behaviors; the utility of stereotype-based scales, especially in predicting everyday behavior; developmental stage needs; social-cognitive aspects; theoretical approaches; and idiographic considerations. All these topics led to greater awareness of the difficulty of knowing a social reality which is co-constructed by all participants and changing over time. The biological, the cognitive, the identity, the social, and the historical aspects of the situation must be addressed in sex-role development research. Studies led to ten important conclusions for sex-role research (presented in the preface and in chapter 5).

A major study of sex roles touching on some of these issues was reported, and methodological issues in using sex-role inventories with older respondents were discussed. We conducted a study of 364 community-dwelling mature adults, aged 60 and over, to determine: (1) whether they generally describe themselves in androgynous sex-role terms or in nonandrogynous terms; (2) whether current life experiences, past milestone events, or perceived social expectations about roles might be related to described sex role, and (3) whether sex-role complexity is associated with successful aging. These research questions were embedded in a theoretical view of sex-role development in which the sex role adopted is adapted to the biological, psychological, social, and environmental contingencies experienced by the individual at a given life stage. Measures included the BSRI; standard assessment of verbal intelligence, mental health, physical health, morale, life event stress; and questions gathering information on milestone events, decision-making, and demographic data.

Results supported most of our hypotheses and led to the following conclusions.

1. A cohort of older adults is primarily androgynous. This hypothesis was confirmed since the majority of the sample tested was androgynous in sex role. Factors obtained from analyses of BSRI responses, while qualitatively different in some respects from factors obtained for younger cohorts, did rotate to similar dimensions. No striking age or sex differences in factors were found.

2. Respondents typed feminine make more visits to health service providers than the androgynous or masculine respondents do. This hypothesis was not supported but its reverse was; i.e. masculine respondents made more visits while feminine made less, even with sex controlled. Perhaps there is a relation between agentic orientation and doctor visits. Health was not a mediator of the relationship described. A new alternative hypothesis, given these findings, might be that doctor visits lead to an agentic orientation, rather than flowing from it.

3. Respondents project a consensus on role attributes expected for older men and older women. This hypothesis was supported.

4. Individuals whose actual roles differ from their perceived socially expected roles respond differently to several measures, including morale and symptomatology. Only symptomatology was a significant factor related to sex-role strain or conflict.

5. Members of sex-type groups report different milestone events, differing recent life events, and differing resolution styles of complex decisions. Results were not clear-cut on this hypothesis. The reader is referred to results sections (chapter 8) that are appropriate for summaries of a number of result patterns relating to this hypothesis.

6. Androgynous elders age more successfully than those of other groups. This hypothesis was supported, but not uniformly across every dimension of successful aging.

The chapter by *Windle* identified a major psychometric issue in the study of development and aging, that of measurement equivalence, and proposed an analytical strategy to deal with it. Data on sex roles and aging were used to illustrate how one might proceed to test alternative hypotheses about the underlying factorial structure of a measure for multiple samples. LISREL-V was introduced and utilized in the assessment of varying degrees of factorial invariance across samples of older adult males and females. Factorial invariance was found for the factor loading patterns and the intercorrelation matrices for the two samples. While the application of CFA was limited to similarities and differences between genders of older adults, it has potential for assessing similarities and differences among age groups and to test theoretical expectations regarding developmental change phenomena.

Caveats for Future Research

Further thought and empirical work in the area of sex-role development in later adulthood is needed as evidenced by comments in earlier chapters of this book. Future work ought to address some of the following questions and issues:

(1) Role stereotypes (positive and negative), role-related behaviors, and gender-linked expectations all must be considered as potentially different phenomena in sex-role research. The nature of test questions themselves is important. The scope, nature, variability, and contextual factors in each must be explored.

(2) Roles must not be assumed to be linked to actual behavior or be predictive of behavior, without evidence.

(3) Role strength must be considered; one can be considered masculine, feminine, or androgynous *only* relative to some standard.

(4) Perceptions, intentions, belief systems, and meanings are important neglected variables in sex-role research.

(5) Sex-role life-span research can be integrated with Piagetian approaches, cognitive research in general, and problem-solving research. It should be.

(6) Sex-role development research should use models of change over time from new physics theories, systems theory, etc., to broaden the repertoire of multivariate approaches at its disposal and better reflect the reality of these complex multisystem changes.

(7) The impact of roles on society and the species and the utility of roles for society and species need to be considered.

(8) Learning and developmental effects need to be considered jointly in future research.

(9) What is adaptive depends on situation, developmental stage, reward and punishment contingencies, past history, and the energy-available state of the person system at a given time.

(10) People have different styles of achieving the same goal or enacting the same intention or reporting the same attitude.

(11) Self-concept, personal continuity, and personal effectiveness are seldom examined but enter into the picture of sex-role development.

(12) Methodological issues need to be clarified, especially including longitudinal research on factor changes. But current approaches still give useful information with careful interpretation.

(13) Tighter theory is needed, preferably from a systems perspective.

(14) Longitudinal studies and studies with behavioral validation need to be performed.

These modest proposals would be beginning steps in the understanding of later stages of sex-role development, an important co-constructed dimension of social 'self' in action.

References

Abrahams, B.; Feldman, S.; Nash, S.: Sex-role self-concept and sex-role attitudes: enduring personality characteristics or adaptations to changing life situations? Devl Psychol. *14:* 393–400 (1978).

Albrecht, S.L.; Bahr, H.M.; Chadwick, B.A.: Changing family and sex roles: an assessment of age differences. J. Marriage Family *41:* 41–50 (1979).

Alpaugh, P.K.; Birren, J.E.: Are there sex differences in creativity across the lifespan? Hum. Dev. *18:* 461–465 (1975).

Alwin, D.F.; Jackson, D.J.: Applications of simultaneous factor analysis to issues of factorial invariance; in Jackson, Borgatta, Factor analysis and measurement in sociological research: a multidimensional perspective (Sage, Beverly Hills 1981).

Ames, L.B.; Learned, J.; Metraux, R.; Walter R.: Rorschach responses in old age (Hoeber, New York 1954).

Ammons, R.B.; Ammons, C.H.: The Quick Test (QT): provisional manual. Psychol. Rep. monogr. suppl. I–VII (1962).

Ammons, R.B.; Ammons, C.H.: Use and evaluation of the Quick Test (QT): partial summary through October 1979. I. Published papers. Psychol. Rep. *45:* 943–946 (1979).

Andersen, S.M.; Bem, S.L.: Sex typing and androgyny in dyadic interaction: individual differences in responsiveness to physical attractiveness. J. Pers. soc. Psychol. *41:* 74–86 (1981).

Antill, J.K.; Cunningham, J.D.: Self-esteem as a function of masculinity in both sexes. J. consult. clin. Psychol. *47:* 783–785 (1979).

Araji, S.K.: Husbands' and wives' attitude-behavior congruence on family roles. J. Marriage Family *39:* 309–320 (1977).

Arieti, S.: Creativity: the magic synthesis (Basic Books, New York 1976).

Bachrach, A.J.: Psychological research (Random House, New York 1981).

Bakan, D.: The duality of human existence (Rand McNally, Chicago 1966).

Bandura, A.; Walters, R.H.: Social learning and personality development (Holt, Rinehart, & Winston, New York 1963).

Barron, F.: Creativity and personal freedom (Van Nostrand, Princeton 1968).

Barrows, G.W.; Zuckerman, M.: Construct validity of three masculinity-femininity tests. J. Counsel. clin. Psychol. *34:* 1–7 (1976).

Barry, H.; Bacon, M.K.; Child, I.L.: A cross-cultural survey of some sex differences in socialization. J. abnorm. soc. Psychol. *55:* 327–332 (1957).

Beauvoir, S. de: The coming of age (Warner, New York 1973).

Beere, C.A.: Women and women's issues, a handbook of tests and measures (Jossey-Bass, San Francisco 1979).

Bell, J.Z.: Disengagement versus engagement – a need for greater expectations. J. Am. Geriat. Soc. *26:* 89–95 (1978).

Bem, S.L.: Measurement of psychological androgyny. J. consult. clin. Psychol. *42:* 155–162 (1974).

Bem, S.L.: Sex-role adaptability: one consequence of psychological androgyny. J. Pers. soc. Psychol. *31:* 634–643 (1975).

Bem, S.L.: Theory and measurement of androgyny: a reply to the Pedhazur-Tetenbaum and Locksley-Colten critiques. J. pers. soc. Psychol. *37:* 1047–1054 (1979).

Bem, S.L.: Gender-schema theory: a cognitive account of sex typing. Psychol. Rev. *88:* 354–364 (1981a).

Bem, S.L.: The BSRI and gender schema theory: a reply to Spence and Helmreich. Psychol. Rev. *88:* 369–371 (1981b).

Bem, S.L.: Gender schema theory and self schema theory compared: a comment on Markus, Crane, Bernstein and Siladi's 'Self-schemas and Gender'. J. Pers. soc. Psychol. *43:* 1192–1194 (1982).

Bem, S.L.; Lenney, E.: Sex typing and the avoidance of cross-sex behavior. J. Pers. soc. Psychol. *33:* 48–54 (1976).

Bem, S.L.; Martyna, W.; Watson, S.: Sex typing and androgyny: further explorations of the expressive domain. J. Pers. soc. Psychol. *34:* 1016–1023 (1976).

Bentler, P.M.: Multivariate analysis with latent variables: causal modeling. A. Rev. Psychol. *31:* 419–456 (1980).

Bernard, J.: Change and stability in sex-role norms and behavior. J. soc. Issues *32:* 207–223 (1976).

Bernard, L.C.: Multivariate analysis of new sex role formulations and personality. J. Pers. soc. Psychol. *38:* 323–336 (1980).

Bertalanfy, L. von: General systems theory (Braziller, New York 1968).

Berzins, J.I.; Welling, M.A.; Wetter, R.E.: The PRF ANDRO scale user's manual (revised); unpublished manuscript, Lexington (1977).

Berzins, J.I.; Welling, M.A.; Wetter, R.E.: A new measure of psychological androgyny based on the Personality Research Form. J. consult. clin. Psychol. *46:* 126–138 (1978).

Bliwise, N.G.; Brown, B.B.; Zindler, M.: Age, gender, and ethnic differences in self-perceived personal changes. Meet. Gerontological Society, San Diego 1980.

Block, J.H.: Conceptions of sex-role. Am. Psychol. *28:* 512–526 (1973).

Braden, B.B.: Dreams for development: midlife perspectives on relational vs individualistic goals; unpublished diss., Garden City (1982).

Breytspraak, L.M.: The development of self in later life (Little, Brown, Boston 1984).

Britton, J.; Britton, J.: Personality changes in aging (Springer, New York 1972).

Buckley, W.: Modern systems research for the behavioral scientist (Aldine, Chicago 1968).

Butler, R.; Lewis, M.: Aging and mental health (Mosby, St Louis 1973).

Cameron, P.: Masculinity/femininity of the generations: as self reported and stereotypically appraised. Int. J. Aging hum. Dev. *7:* 143–151 (1976).

Cherry, D.L.; Zarit, W.H.: Sex-role and age differences in competency, flexibility, and affective status of women; unpublished manuscript (1979).

Clayton, V.: Erikson's theory of human development as it applies to the aged: wisdom as contradictive cognition. Hum. Dev. *18:* 119–128 (1975).

Commons, M.; Richards, F.A.; Armon, C.: Beyond formal operations: late adolescent and adult cognitive development (Praeger, New York 1984).

Constantinople, A.: Masculinity-femininity: an exception to a famous dictum? Psychol. Bull. *80:* 389–407 (1973).

Costa, P.; McCrae, R.: Cross-sectional differences in masculinity and femininity in adult men. Meet. Gerontological Society, San Francisco 1977.

Crane, M.; Markus, H.: Gender identity: the benefits of a self-schema approach. J. Pers. soc. Psychol. *43:* 1195–1197 (1982).

Cureton, E.E.; D'Agostino, R.B.: Factor analysis: an applied approach (Erlbaum, Hillsdale 1983).

Datan, N.; Rodeheaver, D.: Beyond generativity: toward a sensuality of later life: in Weg, Sexuality in the later years (Academic Press, New York 1983).

Davis, L.J.; Brody, E.M.: Rape and older women (NIMH, HEW, Bethesda, Md. 1979).

Deaux, K.: The behavior of women and men (Brooks/Cole, Monterey, Calif. 1976).

De Gregorio, E.; Carver, C.S.: Type-A behavior pattern, sex-role orientation, and psychological adjustment. J. Pers. soc. Psychol. *39:* 286–293 (1980).

Dobzhansky, T.: Genetic diversity and human equality (Basic Books, New York 1973).

Dohrenwend, B.; Dohrenwend, B.S.: Social status and psychological disorder (Wiley, New York 1969).

Douglas, K.; Arenberg, D.: Age changes, cohort differences and cultural change on the Guilford-Zimmerman Temperament Survey. J. Geront. *33:* 737–747 (1978).

Eagley, A.H.; Steffen, V.J.: Gender stereotypes stem from the distributions of women and men into social roles. J. Pers. soc. Psychol. *46:* 735–754 (1984).

Eckensberger, L.H.: Methodological issues of cross-cultural research in developmental psychology; in Nesselroade, Reese, Life-span developmental psychology (Academic Press, New York 1973).

Emmerich, W.: Socialization and sex-role development; in Baltes, Schaie, Life-span developmental psychology: personality and socialization (Academic Press, New York 1973).

Erikson, E.: Childhood and society (Norton, New York 1963).

Evanoski, P.J.; Maher, T.J.: Masculinity, femininity, and psychological well-being. Meet. Am. Psychological Ass., New York 1979.

Foley, J.M.; Murphy, D.M.: Sex-role identity in the aged. Meeting of the Gerontological Society, San Francisco 1977.

Frederiksen, N.: How to tell if a test measures the same things in different cultures; in Poortinga, Basic problems in cross-cultural psychology (Offsetdrukkerij Kanters, 1977).

Freud, S.: Three essays on the theory of sexuality; in Strachey, The standard edition of the complete psychological works of Sigmund Freud, vol. 7 (Hogarth Press/Institute of Psychoanalysis, London 1964; originally published 1905).

Freud, S.: Some psychological consequences of the anatomical distinction between the sexes; in Strachey, Collected papers, vol. 5 (Norton, New York, 1959; originally published 1925).

Frieze, I.H.; Parsons, J.E.; Johnson, P.B.; Ruble, D.N.; Zellman, G.L: Women and sex roles, a social psychological perspective (Norton, New York 1978).

Garnets, L.; Pleck, J.H.: Sex-role identity, androgyny, and sex-role transcendence: a sex-role strain analysis. Psychol. Women Q. *3:* 270–283 (1979).

Gendreau, L.; Roach, T.; Gendreau, P.: Assessing the intelligence of aged persons: report on the Quick Test. Psychol. Rep. *32:* 475–480 (1973).

Gillett, N.; Levitt, M.; Antonucci, T.: The relationship between masculinity, femininity, and social competence in three generations of women. Meet. Gerontological Society, San Francisco 1977.

Gilligan, C.: In a different voice (Harvard University Press, Cambridge 1982).

Gorsuch, R.L.: Factor analysis; 2nd ed. (Erlbaum, Hillsdale 1983).

Gove, W.R.: Sex, marital status, and suicide. J. Health soc. Issues *13:* 204–213 (1972a).

Gove, W.R.: The relationship between sex roles, marital status, and mental illness. Soc. Forces *51:* 34–44 (1972b).

Gove, W.R.; Geerkin, M.R.: The effect of children and employment on the mental health of married men and women. Soc. Forces *56:* 66–76 (1977).

Gross, A.E.: The male role and heterosexual behavior. J. soc. Issues *34:* 87–107 (1978).

Gutmann, D.: Parenthood: a key to the comparative study of the life cycle; in Datan, Ginsberg, Life-span developmental psychology: normative crises (Academic Press, New York 1975).

Gutmann, D.: The parental imperative revisited: towards a developmental psychology of adulthood and later life; in Meacham, Family and individual development (Karger, Basel 1985).

Gutmann, D.; Grunes, J.; Griffin, B.: The clinical psychology of later life: developmental paradigms. Meet. Gerontological Society, Washington 1979.

Guttentag, M.; Secord, P.F.: Too many women? The sex ratio question (Sage, Beverly Hills 1983).

Guttmann, D.; Sinnott, J.D.; Carrigan, Z.; Holahan, N.; Flynn, M.; Mullaney, J.: The impact of needs, knowledge, ability, and living arrangements on decision-making of the elderly (Catholic University Press, Washington 1977).

Hancock, K.A.: A study of locus of control and psychological androgyny in women as a function of age and feminism; unpublished, doct. diss., California School of Professional Psychology (1978).

Harlow, H.F.: The nature of love. Am. Psychol. *13:* 673–685 (1958).

Harrison, J.: Warning: the male sex-role may be dangerous to your health; in Pleck, Brannon, Male roles and male experience. J. soc. Issues *34:* 65–86 (1978).

Havighurst, R.J.: Human development and education (McCay, New York 1953).

Hefner, R.; Rebecca, M.; Oleshansky, B.: Development of sex-role transcendence. Hum. Dev. *18:* 143–158 (1975).

Heilbrun, A.B.: An exploration of antecedents and attributes of androgynous and undifferentiated sex roles. J. genet. Psychol. *132:* 97–107 (1978).

Helson, H.: Adaptation level theory (Harper & Row, New York 1964).

Hoffman, D.M.; Fidell, L.S.: Characteristics of androgynous, undifferentiated masculine and feminine middle-class women. Sex Roles *5:* 765–781 (1979).

Hofstadter, D.R.: Gödel, Esher, Bach: an eternal golden braid (Vintage Books, New York 1979).

Holmes, T.H.; Masuda, M.: Life changes and illness susceptibility; in Dohrenwend, Dohrenwend, Stressful life events, their nature and effects (Wiley & Sons, New York 1964).

Homes, T.H.; Rahe, R.H.: The social readjustment rating scale. J. psychomat. Res. *11:* 213–218 (1967).

Hubbard, R.W.; Santos, J.F.; Farrow, B.J.: Age differences in sex-role diffusion: a study of middle-aged and older adult married couples. Meet. Gerontological Society, Washington 1979.

Inhelder, B.; Piaget, J.: The growth of logical thinking from childhood to adolescence (Basic Books, New York 1958).

Jackson, D.N.: Personality Research Form Manual (Research Psychologists Press, New York 1967).

Jacobson, D.: The effects of selected personal-social factors on cognitive functioning in the aging; doct. diss., Washington (1974).

James, L.R.; Mulaik, S.A.; Brett, J.M.: Causal analysis: assumptions, models, and data (Sage Publications, Beverly Hills 1982).

Jewett, S.: Longevity and the longevity syndrome. Gerontologist *13:* 91–99 (1973).

Jöreskog, K.G.: Simultaneous factor analysis in several populations. Psychometrika *36:* 409–426 (1971).

Jöreskog, K.G.; Sorbom, D.: EFAP-II exploratory factor analysis program (National Educational Resources, Chicago 1978).

Jöreskog, K.G.; Sorbom, D.: Advances in factor analysis and structural equation models (Abt Books, Cambridge 1979).

Jöreskog, K.G.; Sorbom, D.: LISREL V: analysis of linear structural relationships by maximum likelihood and least squares methods (National Education Resources, Chicago 1981).

Jung, C.G.: Modern men in search of a soul (Research Psychologists Press, New York 1933).

Kagan, J.: Acquisition and significance of sex-typing and sex-role identity; in Hoffman, Hoffman, Review of child development research (Sage, New York 1964).

Kelly, G.A.: The psychology of personal constructs (Norton, New York 1955).

Kelly, J.A.; Worell, J.: New formulations of sex roles and androgyny: a critical review. J. consult. Clin. Psychol. *45:* 1101–1115 (1977).

Kline, C.: The socialization process of women. Gerontologist *15:* 486–492 (1975).

Kohlberg, L.: A cognitive-developmental analysis of children's sex-role concepts and attitudes; in Maccoby, The development of sex differences (Stanford University Press, Stanford 1966).

Kramer, D.: Postformal operations? A need for further conceptualization. Hum. Dev. *26:* 91–105 (1983).

Kuhn, T.S.: The structure of scientific revolutions (University of Chicago Press, Chicago 1962).

Labouvie, E.W.: Identity versus equivalence of psychological measures and constructs; in Poon, Aging in the 1980s: selected contemporary issues in the psychology of aging (Am. Psychological Ass., Washington 1980).

Labouvie-Vief, G.: Beyond formal operations: uses and limits of pure logic in life-span development. Hum. Dev. *23:* 141–161 (1980).

La France, M.; Carmen, B.: The nonverbal display of psychological androgyny. J. Pers. soc. Psychol. *38:* 36–49 (1980).

Langner, T.A.: A twenty-two item screening score of psychiatric symptoms indicating impairment. J. Hlth soc. Behav. *3:* 269–276 (1962).

Lawton, M.P.: The Philadelphia Geriatric Morale Scale: a revision. J. Geront. *30:* 85–89 (1975).

Lenny, E.: Androgyny: some audacious assertions toward its coming of age. Sex roles *5:* 703–719 (1979a).

Lenny, E.: Concluding comments on androgyny: some limitations of its mature development. Sex Roles *5:* 829 (1979b).

Levine, N.: Validation of the Quick Test for intelligence screening of the elderly. Psychol. Rep. *29:* 167–172 (1971).

Lewis, R.A.: Emotional intimacy among men; in Pleck, Brannon, Male roles and the male experience. J. soc. Issues *34:* 108–121 (1978).

Livson, F.B.: Patterns of personality development in middle-aged women: a longitudinal study. Int. J. Aging hum. Devl. *7:* 107–115 (1976).

Livson, F.B.: Gender identity: a lifespan view of sex-role development; in Weg, Sexuality in the later years: roles and behavior (Academic Press, New York 1983).

Locksley, A.; Colten M.E.: Psychological androgyny: a case of mistaken identity? J. Pers. soc. Psychol. *37:* 1017–1031 (1979).

Loevinger, J.: Ego development (Jossey-Bass, San Francisco 1977).

Looft, C.: Socialization and personality throughout the life span: an examination of contemporary psychological approaches; in Baltes, Schaie, Life-span developmental psychology: personality and socialization (Academic Press, New York 1973).

Lowenthal, M.F.; Thurnher, M.; Chriboga, D.: Four stages of life: a comparative study of women and men facing transition (Jossey-Bass, San Francisco 1975)

Lumsden, C.J.; Wilson, E.O.: Genes, mind, and culture: a coevolutionary process (Harvard University Press, Cambridge 1981).

Maccoby, E.; Jacklin, C.: The psychology of sex differences (Stanford University Press, Stanford 1974).

Manis, J.: The sociology of knowledge and community mental health research. Soc. Problems *15:* 488–501 (1968).

Manning, T.T.: Sex-typed and androgynous males and females: personality and ego development differences (Am. Psychological Ass., San Francisco 1977).

Maslow, A.H.: Religion, values, and peak experiences (Ohio State University Press, Columbus 1964).

McGee, J.; Wells, K.: Gender typing and androgyny in later life: new directions for theory and research. Hum. Dev. *25:* 116–139 (1982).

Mead, M.: Sex and temperament in three primitive societies (Morrow, New York 1935).

Mechanic, D.: Sociocultural and social-psychological factors affecting personal responses to psychological disorders. J. Hlth soc. Behav. *16:* 393–404 (1975).

Merchant, C.: The death of nature (Harper & Row, San Francisco 1982).

Miller, J.: Living systems (McGraw-Hill, New York 1978).

Mills, C.J.; Tyrrell, D.J.: Sex stereotypic encoding and release from proactive interference. J. Pers. soc. Psychol. *45:* 772–781 (1983).

Mischel, W.: Sex-typing and socialization; in Mussen, Carmichael's manual of child psychology, vol. 2 (Wiley, New York 1970).

Money, J.; Ehrhardt, A.A.: Man and woman, boy and girl: the differentiation and dimorphism of gender identity from conception to maturity (Johns Hopkins University Press, Baltimore 1972).

Moreland, J.R.; Harren, V.A.; Krimsky-Montague, E.; Tinsley, E.A.: Sex-role self-concept and career decision making. J. Counsel. Psychol. *26:* 329–336 (1979).

Mulaik, S.: The foundations of factor analysis (McGraw-Hill, New York 1972).

Murphy, D.M.: Sex-role identity in the aged; doct. diss., Chicago (1976).

Muthen, B.: A general structural equation model with dichotomous, ordered categorical, and continuous latent variable indicators. Psychometrika *49:* 115–132 (1984).

Neugarten, B: Personality in middle and late life (Prentice-Hall, New York 1964).

Neugarten, B. (ed.): Middle age and aging (University of Chicago Press, Chicago 1968).

Neugarten, B.; Crotty, G.; Tobin, S.: Personality types in an aging population; in Neugarten, Personality in middle and late life (Prentice Hall, New York 1964).

Neugarten, B.; Gutmann, D.: Age-sex roles and personality in middle age: a TAT study; in Neugarten, Middle age and aging (University of Chicago Press, Chicago 1968).

Neugarten, B.; Havighurst, R.; Tobin, S.: Personality and patterns of aging; in Neugarten, Middle age and aging (University of Chicago Press, Chicago 1968).

O'Sullivan, W.M.: A study of the relationship between life satisfaction of the aged and perceptions they hold concerning their own masculinity and femininity; doct. diss., New York (1980).

Palmore, E.: Differences in the retirement patterns of men and women. Gerontologist 5: 4–8 (1965).

Parsons, T.; Bales, R.: Family, socialization, and interaction process (Free Press, New York 1955).

Petersen, A.C.: Biophysical processes in the development of sex-related differences; in Parsons, The psychobiology of sex differences and sex roles (Hemisphere, Washington 1980).

Peterson, L.M.: Self-esteem and sex type: a function of the scale? Meet. Eastern Psychological Ass., New York 1981.

Piaget, J.: The moral judgement of the child (Free Press of Glencoe, New York 1948).

Piaget, J.; Kamii, C.: What is psychology? Am. Psychol. 33: 648–652 (1978).

Pleck, J.H.: The male sex role: definitions, problems, and sources of change. J. soc. Issues 32: 155–164 (1976).

Prigogene, I.: From being to becoming (Freeman, San Francisco 1980).

Prigogene, I.; Stengers, I.: Order out of chaos, man's new dialogue with nature (Bantam, New York 1984).

Puglisi, J.T.; Jackson, D.W.: Sex-role identity and self-esteem in adulthood. Int. J. Aging hum. Devl. 12: 129–138 (1980–81).

Reichard, S.; Livson, F.; Peterson, P.: Aging and personality (Wiley, New York 1962).

Richardson, M.S.; Merrifield, P.; Jacobson, A.: A factor analytic study of the Bem Sex-Role Inventory. Meet. Am. Psychological Ass., New York 1979.

Riegel, K.F.: Dialectical operations: the final period of human development. Hum. Dev. 16: 346–370 (1973).

Riegel, K.F.: Toward a dialectical theory of development. Hum. Dev. 18: 50–64 (1975).

Riegel, K.F.: The dialectics of human development. Am. Psychol. 31: 679–700 (1976).

Sanday, P.R.: Female power and male dominance (Cambridge University Press, Cambridge 1981).

Schaie, K.W.: Quasi-experimental research designs in the psychology of aging; in Birren, Schaie, Handbook of the psychology of aging (Van Nostrand & Reinhold, New York 1977).

Schaie, K.W.; Schaie, J.P.: Clinical assessment and aging; in Birren, Schaie, Handbook of the psychology of aging (Van Nostrand & Reinhold, New York 1977).

Sedney, M.A.: Process of sex-role development during life crises of middle-aged women. Meet. Gerontological Society, San Francisco 1977.

Senneker, P.; Hendrick, C.: Androgyny and helping behavior. J. Pers. soc. Psychol. 45: 916–925 (1983).

Shields, S.: Functionalism, Darwinism, and the psychology of women. Am. Psychol. *30:* 739–754 (1975).

Silverman, M.: The old man as woman: detecting stereotypes of aged men with a femininity scale. Percept. Mot. Skills *44:* 336–338 (1977).

Silvern, L.E.; Ryan, V.L.: Self-rated adjustment and sex typing on the Bem Sex-Role Inventory: Is masculinity the primary predictor of adjustment? Sex Roles *5:* 739–763 (1979).

Sinnott, J.D.: Everyday thinking and Piagetian operativity in adults. Hum. Dev. *18:* 430–443 (1975).

Sinnott, J.D.: Sex-role inconstancy, biology, and successful aging: a dialectical model. Gerontologist *17:* 459–463 (1977).

Sinnott, J.D.: Adult intellectual development as social-cognitive growth: a model. Meet. Gerontological Society, Dallas 1978.

Sinnott, J.D.: The theory of relativity: a metatheory for development? Hum. Dev. *24:* 293–311 (1981).

Sinnott, J.D.: Correlates of sex roles in older adults. J. Geront. *37:* 587–594 (1982).

Sinnott, J.D.: A model for solutions of ill-structured problems: implications for everyday and abstract problem solving. Meet. Gerontological Society, San Francisco 1983.

Sinnott, J.D.: Older men, older women, are their perceived sex roles similar? Sex Roles *10:* 847–856 (1984a).

Sinnott, J.D.: Postformal reasoning: the relativistic stage; in Commons, Richards, Armon, Beyond formal operations (Praeger, New York 1984b).

Sinnott, J.D.: Sex, health, and mental health of older women and men. Int. J. Aging hum. Dev. *20:* 123–132 (1984c).

Sinnott, J.D.; Block, M.R.; Grambs, J.D.; Gaddy, C.D.; Davidson, J.L.: Sex roles in mature adults: antecedents and correlates (Center on Aging, University of Maryland, College Park 1980).

Sinnott, J.D.; Guttmann, D.: Piagetian logical abilities and older adults' abilities to solve everyday problems. Hum. Dev. *21:* 327–333 (1978a).

Sinnott, J.D.; Guttmann, D.: The dialectics of decision-making and older adults. Hum. Dev. *21:* 190–200 (1978b).

Skinner, R.J.: Relationship between sex-role identity and perceived health in elderly females; doct. diss., Austin (1979).

Smith, M.Y.: Impact of age and environment on gender roles among S.R.O. elderly; doct. diss., Lafayette (1981).

Spence, J.T.; Helmreich, R.L.: Masculinity and femininity: their psychological dimensions, correlates, and antecedents (University of Texas Press, Austin 1978).

Spence, J.T.; Helmreich, R.L.: Comparison of masculine and feminine personality attributes and sex-role attitudes across age groups. Devl. Psychol. *15:* 583–584 (1979a).

Spence, J.T.; Helmreich, R.L.: On assessing 'androgyny'. Sex Roles *5:* 721–738 (1979b).

Spence, J.T.; Helmreich, R.; Stapp, J.: The Personal Attributes Questionnaire: a measure of sex-role stereotypes and masculinity-femininity. JSAS Catalog of Selected Documents in Psychology *4:* 43–44 (1974).

Spence, J.T.; Helmreich, R.; Stapp, J.: Ratings of self and peers on sex-role attitudes and their relation to self-esteem and conceptions of masculinity and femininity. J. Pers. soc. Psychol. *32:* 29–39 (1975).

Storms, M.D.: Sex-role identity and its relation to sex-role attributes and sex-role stereotypes. J. Pers. soc. Psychol. *37:* 1779–1789 (1979).

Strahan, R.F.: Remarks on Bem's measurement of psychological adrogyny: alternative methods and a supplementary analysis. J. consult. Clin. Psych. *43:* 568–571 (1975).

Suzuki, T.F.: A conceptual analysis of sex-role identity and its interaction with gender and chronological age; doct. diss., Gainesville (1979).

Tanner, N.M.: On becoming human (Cambridge University Press, Cambridge 1981).

Tavris, C.; Offir, C.: The longest war, sex differences in perspective (Harcourt Brace & Jovanovich, New York 1977).

Taylor, M.C.; Hall, J.A.: Psychological androgyny: theories, methods, conclusions. Psychol. Bull. *92:* 347–366 (1982).

Toffler, A.: Future shock (Bantam, New York 1970).

Toffler, A.: The third wave (Bantam, New York 1980).

Turner, B.F.: Sex roles among wives in middle and late life. Convention of the Am. Psychological Ass., San Francisco 1977.

Uleman, J.S.; Weston, M.: Changing social roles changes BSRI masculinity and femininity. Meet. Eastern Psychological Ass., Baltimore 1984.

Urberg, K.A.: Sex role conceptualizations in adolescents and adults. Devl Psych. *15:* 90–92 (1979).

Vale, J.R.: Genes, environment, and behavior (Harper & Row, New York 1980).

Weg, R.B.: Sexuality in the later years (Academic Press, New York 1983).

Wells, K.: Towards a model of gender-role development in adulthood: the transition from gender-typing to androgyny. Association for Women in Psychology Conf., Dallas 1979.

Whelton, C.; Swindells, T.: A factor analysis of the Bem Sex-Role Inventory. J. clin. Psychol. *33:* 150–153 (1977).

Whitley, B.E.: Sex-role self-concept and self-esteem: a critical meta-analytic review. Meet. Eastern Psychological Ass., New York 1981.

Williams, R.; Wirth, C.: Lives through the years (Atherton Press, New York 1965).

Windle, M.: Sex-role orientation, cognitive flexibility, and life satisfaction among older adults. Psychol. Women Q. (in press, 1986).

Windle, M.; Sinnott, J.D.: A psychometric study of the Bem Sex-Role Inventory with an older adult sample. J. Geront. *40:* 336–343 (1985).

Wish, C.W.: The relationship of sex-role typing to life satisfaction in older persons; doct. diss., Columbus (1976).

Wolf, F.A.: Taking the quantum leap (Harper & Row, New York 1981).

Wood, P.K.: Inquiring systems and problem structure. Hum. Devl. *26:* 249–265 (1983).

Worell, J.: Androgyny and psychological well-being: some ideological dilemmas. Meet. Society for Research in Child Development, Boston 1981.

Zaks, P.M.; Karuza, J.; Domurath, K.L.; Labouvie-Vief, G.: Sex-role orientation across the adult life-span. Meet. Gerontological Society, Washington 1979.

Author Index

Subject Index

Action 13, 25 ff., 116, 121
Adaptation 13, 15, 18, 25 ff., 54, 60, 93, 97, 101, 121
Adult development 7 ff., 22, 43 ff., 55
Agency 29 ff., 81
Aging 18, 19, 43 ff., 57 ff.
Attitudes 1, 51

Bem Sex-Role Inventory (BSRI) 35 ff., 60, 66 ff., 74, 93, 103 ff.
Biology 5, 21, 28, 57, 59, 93, 97

Cognitive development 5, 11 ff., 40, 55, 58, 99, 121
Communion 29 ff., 81
Conflict, *see* Roles
Coping 21, 66, 70, 82, 92, 93, 97
Creativity 21, 52
Culture 2, 22, 34, 93, 97, 117, 121

Dialectical theory 2, 18 ff., 22, 71, 99

Education 1, 65, 81, 95
Environment 1 ff., 26, 28, 33, 37 ff., 93 ff.
Expectations, *see* Roles

Feminity 4, 10, 35 ff., 66 ff., 76, 97, 103 ff.

Future shock 25 ff.

Health 23, 47, 61, 66, 71, 81, 92, 95
Humanism 39, 120

Individual differences 121
Instinct 27
Intelligence 60, 66, 69 ff., 81, 95

Learning 3, 21, 27, 43, 45, 58, 85
Life
    events 40, 45, 47, 49, 52, 58, 67, 70, 85, 90, 92
    satisfaction 20, 47, 50, 51, 60, 63, 66, 71, 92
Life-span approach 8, 22, 39, 57
Living systems, *see* Systems theory

Masculinity 4, 10, 35 ff., 66 ff., 76, 97, 103 ff.
Measurement 9 ff., 35 ff., 44, 53, 54, 66, 72 ff., 76 ff., 103 ff., 121
Mental health 23, 37, 47, 49, 60, 61, 66, 72, 81, 90, 92, 95

Oedipal conflict 3